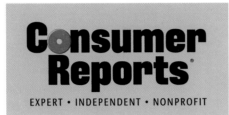

EXPERT • INDEPENDENT • NONPROFIT

2005 Guide to

Diet, Health & Fitness

Consumer Reports

EXPERT • INDEPENDENT • NONPROFIT

2005 Guide to Diet, Health & Fitness

TIME INC. HOME ENTERTAINMENT:

President Rob Gursha
Vice President, New Product Development Richard Fraiman
Executive Director, Marketing Service Carol Pittard
Director, Retail & Special Sales Tom Mifsud
Director of Finance Tricia Griffin
Director, New Product Development Peter Harper
Marketing Director Ann Marie Doherty
Prepress Manager Emily Rabin
Book Production Manager Jonathan Polsky
Special thanks to: Bozena Bannett, Alexandra Bliss, Bernadette Corbie, Robert Dente, Anne-Michelle Gallero, Suzanne Janso, Robert Marasco, Natalie McCrea, Brooke McGuire, Margarita Quiogue, Mary Jane Rigoroso, Steven Sandonato.

TIME INC.

1271 Avenue of the Americas
New York, NY 10020

ISBN: 1-932273-38-7

Time Inc. Home Entertainment is a trademark of Time Inc.

We welcome your comments and suggestions about Time Inc. Books. Please write to us at: Time Inc. Books, Attention: Book Editors, PO Box 11016, Des Moines, IA 50336-1016.

If you would like to order more copies of this book, please call us at 1-800-327-6388. (Monday through Friday, 7:00 a.m.-8:00 p.m. or Saturday, 7:00 a.m.-6:00 p.m. Central Time).

> The information presented in this book is in no way intended to be a substitute for medical care and advice. This book is solely for information and educational purposes. Please consult a medical or health professional before you begin any new exercise or nutrition program or if you have questions about your health.

CONSUMER REPORTS:

President James Guest
Executive Vice President Joel Gurin
Vice President/Editorial Director Elizabeth Crow
Vice President/Publishing John Sateja
Editor, Consumer Reports/Senior Director Margot Slade
Senior Director/General Manager, Products and Market Development Paige Amidon
Product Manager, Retail Products Carol Lappin
Associate Editorial Director Christine Arrington
Design Director George Arthur
Creative Director Timothy LaPalme
Publishing Operations Director David Fox
Production Associate Letitia Hughes

CONSUMER REPORTS, Health:

Director/Editor Ronni Sandroff
Deputy Editor Ronald Buchheim
Group Managing Editor Nancy Crowfoot
Managing Editor Sue Byrne
Senior Editors Nancy Metcalf, Doug Podolsky
Contributing Editors Teresa Carr, Joel Keehn
Medical Editor Marvin M. Lipman, M.D.
Senior Researcher Christopher Hendel
Editorial Associate Jamie Kopf
Research Associate Ano Lobb

Produced by
SHORELINE PUBLISHING GROUP LLC

President / Editorial Director James Buckley, Jr.
Editor, *Diet, Health & Fitness* Bob Woods
Designer Bill Madrid
Photo Research Dawn Friedman, Viju Mathew

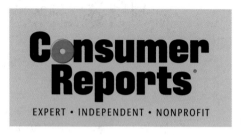

2005 Guide to
Diet, **Health** & **Fitness**

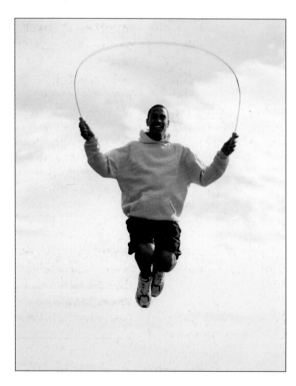

Table of Contents

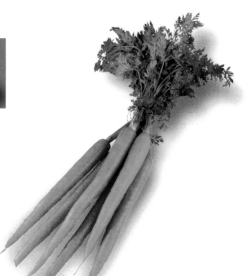

Diet & Nutrition 8-31

Vitamins & Supplements 32-67

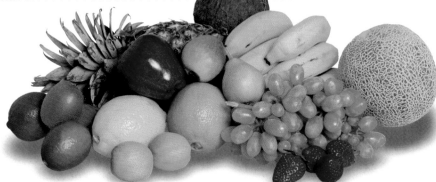

Fitness & Exercise 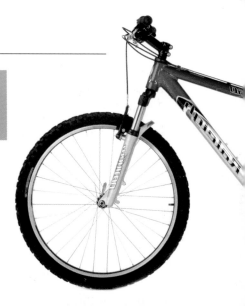 68-93

Health & Wellness 94-171

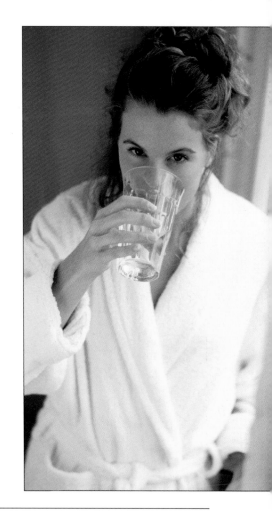

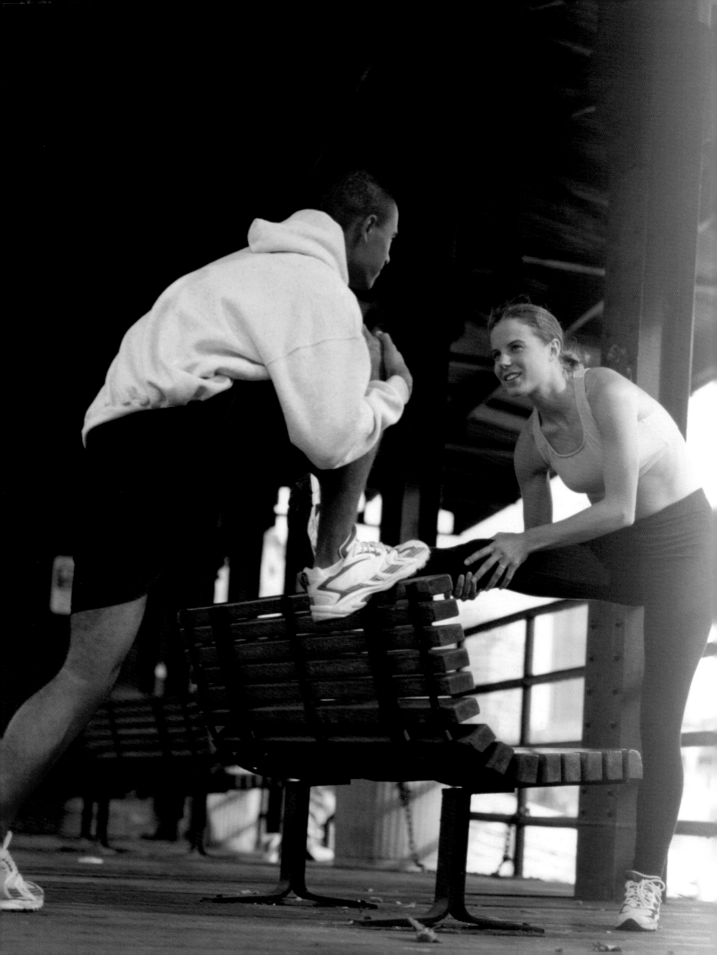

Here's to your health!

In today's fast-paced world, it's a daily challenge to eat right, stay fit, and generally remain happy and healthy. We're bombarded with conflicting advice about which foods, vitamins, and supplements to choose and which ones to avoid; what methods and machines can help us get enough exercise; and which products and services can really assist us in achieving our important health goals. Despite all the hype and promises, too often we're left wondering exactly what to do and who to trust in the process.

This CONSUMER REPORTS *Diet, Health & Fitness Guide* sifts through the clutter in an attempt to provide clear, honest answers. We've compiled the latest articles, surveys, reports, ratings, and recommendations from the editors of CONSUMER REPORTS and its CONSUMER REPORTS on Health monthly newsletter.

The material is conveniently grouped into four sections, each one including hot topics affecting some aspect of your well-being. For example, in Diet & Nutrition, "The truth about dieting" features results from a landmark CONSUMER REPORTS survey, which found that eating filling foods and not skimping on protein are the best solutions for successful weight loss. In "The new, healthier fast food," we explore how the the fast-food industry is making progress in responding to consumers' concerns about excess fats, carbohydrates, and calories.

The Vitamins & Supplements section opens with a troubling report, "Dangerous supplements," about the "dirty dozen" dangerous supplements that CONSUMER REPORTS investigators found still on the market. On a more positive note, "Omega-3 oil: fish or pills?" tells how certain omega-3 fatty acids, from both fish and supplements, can help prevent cardiovascular disease.

We analyze and rate a wide variety of bicycles and treadmills in separate reviews within the Fitness & Exercise section, using the comprehensive Ratings charts that have become a signature of CONSUMER REPORTS over the years. (Be sure to read the notes on each chart, explaining how it was compiled and the range of criteria considered.) "Make the most of your exercise minutes" describes several smart, gentle, and interesting methods that can help even the least-fit individuals achieve their exercise goals.

Among the key topics covered in Health & Wellness are ways to battle high cholesterol, including increasingly prescribed drug treatments, how to keep your immune system strong enough to reduce the risk of serious illness and disease, and how to stay safe in the hospital, a report that examined the experiences—good and bad—of more than 21,000 CONSUMER REPORTS readers.

As with all CONSUMER REPORTS publications, the information in the CONSUMER REPORTS *Diet, Health & Fitness Guide* is presented in a reliable and unbiased manner, intended to keep you up to date. We hope it serves you well. ●

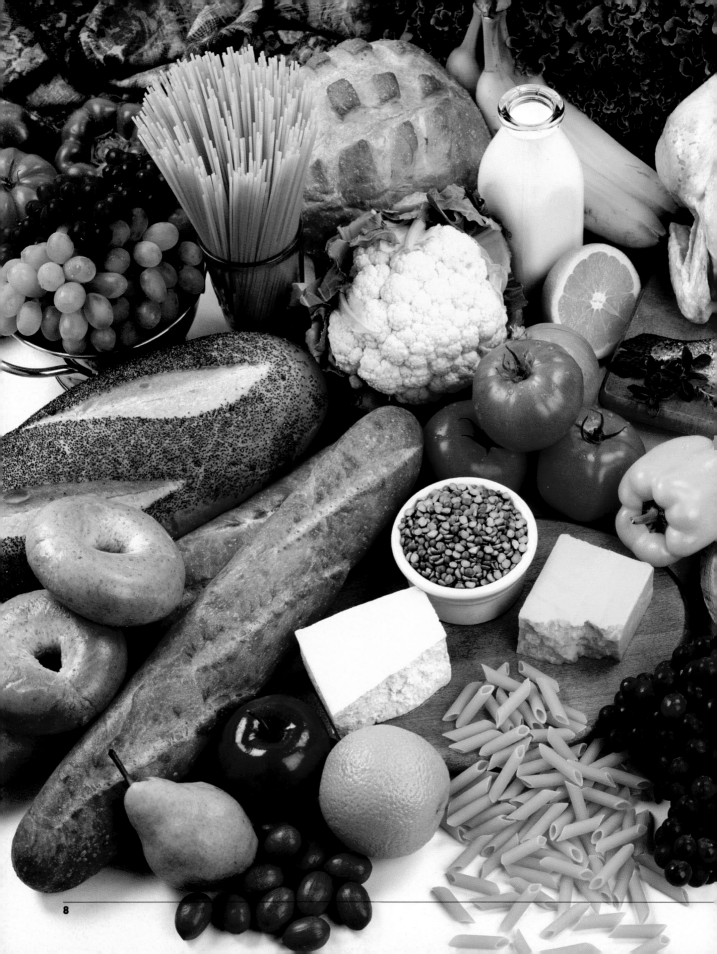

Diet & Nutrition

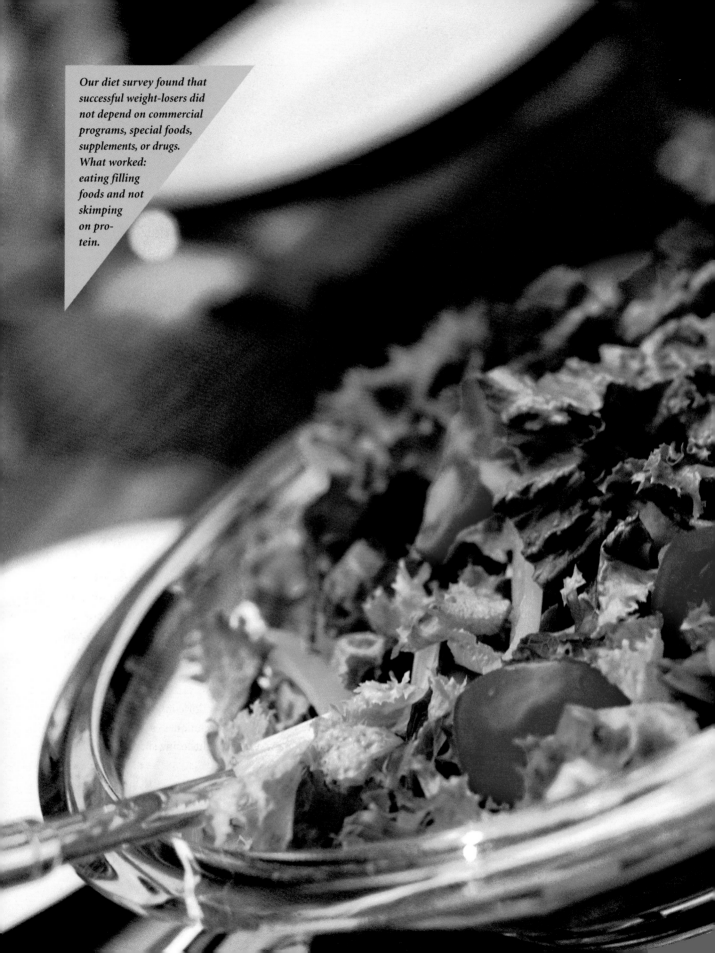

Our diet survey found that successful weight-losers did not depend on commercial programs, special foods, supplements, or drugs. What worked: eating filling foods and not skimping on pro- tein.

The truth about dieting

Fresh veggies fill you up with fiber, water, and disease-fighting nutrients.

In the past decade, Americans have had—and used—every excuse not to diet. Losing weight, they reasoned, is almost impossible unless, like Oprah, you hire your own personal chef and trainer. In an environment where snacks and sweets are constant temptations, a strict low-fat regimen will keep you hungry and miserable for the rest of your life, right?

And even if you do manage to take off all that weight, there's small hope of keeping it off, since studies have shown that 95 percent of all dieters regain their lost weight and go on to add more pounds. When you add it all up, well, praise the Lord and pass the mashed potatoes.

That picture, however, turns out to be overly bleak, according to recent CONSUMER REPORTS research. In the largest survey ever undertaken on the long-term maintenance of weight loss, we found that ordinary people can and do succeed without using expensive commercial diet programs, special foods, dietary supplements, or drugs. Nearly a quarter of the 32,213 dieters who answered our questionnaire lost at least 10 percent of their starting weight and kept it off for at least a year, a standard definition of weight-loss success.

While 25 percent may not be the resounding accomplishment that physicians and nutritionists would want in a nation where one in five adults is obese, it is significant enough to conclude that weight loss is not a hopeless quest. Indeed, among our "losers" were more than 4,000 superlosers who maintained their loss—an average of 37 pounds and often much more than 10 percent of their starting weight—for five years or more.

This news comes at an auspicious time for weight-loss research in general. Scientists are finally addressing an obvious issue they had ignored for years—the hard-wired inability of human beings to tolerate hunger for more than a few days or weeks at a stretch. Their research shows that by following a weight-loss program with a little give in it—one with lean protein and judicious quantities of healthful fats—it's possible to control calorie intake without feeling intolerably hungry. Those techniques, it turns out, were followed by many of our weight-losing successes.

Our survey also showed what you already suspected: Keeping weight off requires regular and fairly rigorous exercise. Eight out of 10 of our successful losers who tried exercising three or more times a week listed it as their No. 1 strategy. And while most chose walking as the path to long-term weight-loss success, an eyebrow-raising 29 percent added weight lifting to their regime.

"This study says that people are succeeding at weight loss by conscious effort," says James Hill, Ph.D., director of the Center for Human Nutrition at the University of Colorado in Denver. "It can be done, but it's not easy. Our challenge is to take what we've learned from these people and use it to help others be successful."

TAKING IT OFF

To find out how well average people do on their diets, we targeted survey respondents who tried to lose weight deliberately. To try to exclude people with eating disorders from our study, we left out dieters who didn't start with a moderately high body mass index, or BMI, of at least 27, a standard measure of fatness that takes into account both height and weight. (For instructions on how to calculate yours, see "Calculate your BMI," on facing page.)

Of our respondents, nearly 8,000 had managed to lose at least 10 percent of their starting weight and keep it off for a year or more. Such a loss won't turn most Americans into runway models, but studies show it can produce dramatic changes in weight-related health conditions such as diabetes and high blood pressure. Among successful dieters with those medical conditions, more than two-thirds said they and their doctors agreed that their condition had improved as a result of the loss.

The best diet strategies help you control calorie intake without feeling hungry.

Strength-training helps replace body fat with muscle.

The superlosers among them—nearly 13 percent of all the dieters—had managed to keep at least 10 percent of their top weight off for five years or more. At their heaviest, 62 percent of this group had been obese, with a BMI of 30 or more and at high risk for weight-related health disorders such as heart disease and high blood pressure. Indeed, about a quarter said they had already developed such problems.

THEY DID IT THEIR WAY

What explains the success of our winning losers? To find out, we compared responses of the 4,056 superstars in our sample—the ones who'd kept their weight off for five years or more—with those of the 3,877 self-admitted failures—people who had tried to lose weight but had shed none at all.

The strongest finding that emerges from the responses, other than the necessity for exercise, is that when it comes to losing weight, one size definitely does not fit all. Eighty-three percent of the successful losers said they lost weight entirely on their own.

That overturns the long-held conviction that to lose weight, you have to enroll in an expensive program, buy special food, or follow the regimen of a particular diet guru. Indeed, just 14 percent of our superlosers had ever signed up with Weight Watchers, Jenny Craig, or other commercial diet programs, while 26 percent of our failures had done so. Eighty-eight percent of our superlosers shunned meal replacements such as Slim Fast. And a mere 6 percent of the successes used dietary supplements or nonprescription weight-loss aids such as Metabolife or Dexatrim. If anything made a difference for them, it was one-on-one counseling from a professional such as a psychologist or nutritionist. Although less than 10 percent of all our 8,000 successes used one, they ranked it second in effectiveness after "my own diet and exercise regimen."

Diets that work match an individual's personal needs and preferences. John Uebersax, 50, a San Diego biostatistician, has maintained a 24-pound weight loss for 12 years by taking brisk walks during work breaks and by follow-

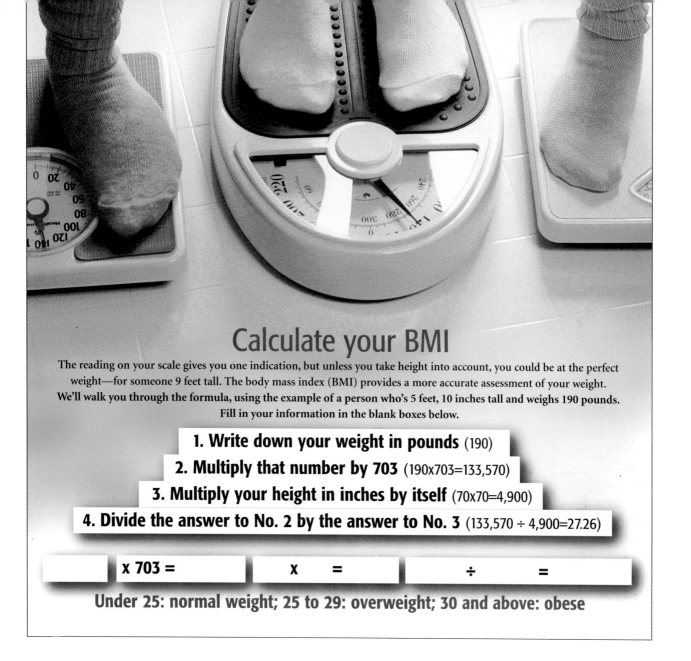

Calculate your BMI

The reading on your scale gives you one indication, but unless you take height into account, you could be at the perfect weight—for someone 9 feet tall. The body mass index (BMI) provides a more accurate assessment of your weight. We'll walk you through the formula, using the example of a person who's 5 feet, 10 inches tall and weighs 190 pounds. Fill in your information in the blank boxes below.

1. Write down your weight in pounds (190)

2. Multiply that number by 703 (190x703=133,570)

3. Multiply your height in inches by itself (70x70=4,900)

4. Divide the answer to No. 2 by the answer to No. 3 (133,570 ÷ 4,900=27.26)

| | x 703 = | | X | = | | ÷ | = |

Under 25: normal weight; 25 to 29: overweight; 30 and above: obese

ing a regimen that evolved in part from a career entailing frequent travel without access to a refrigerator, much less a kitchen. His staples include protein bars, canned tuna, vegetarian meat substitutes, yogurt, fruit, peanuts, and sunflower seeds. He also swallows a spoonful of olive oil each morning. Uebersax says that this unconventional meal plan works fine for him. "I don't like cooking," he says. "I'm not a good cook, and I hate cleaning up."

THE GROWLING STOMACH

Weight loss is no mystery. You have to take in fewer calories than your body burns. "The trick is to help people not feel hungry all the time while they're doing that," says Barbara Rolls, Ph.D., a professor of nutrition at Pennsylvania State University in University Park. Until recently, however, medical researchers mostly aimed at developing diets to achieve medical goals—lowering cholesterol and blood pressure, for example. "We're beginning to say that may not be so great if you won't stay on the diet and you won't be happy," says Adam Drewnowski, Ph.D., director of the nutritional sciences program at the University of Washington in Seattle.

Though obesity experts are still debating the full significance of some of their latest research findings,

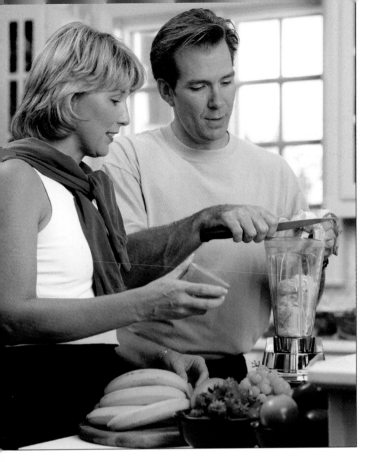

Mixing up a tasty smoothie can help you get your daily 2-4 servings of fruit. Add low-fat yogurt for a dairy requirement.

they've already come up with useful approaches that loser wannabes can apply immediately. Most match the strategies used by the weight-loss achievers who answered our survey:

1. Tame your blood sugar.

The body's use of carbohydrates seems to be key to success. Carbohydrates are the staple of everyday diets, and as much as 55 to 60 percent of the traditional low-fat reducing diet. In the digestive process, carbs break down into glucose (sugar) molecules, which are then sent into the bloodstream. In response to the upsurge in blood sugar, the pancreas secretes the hormone insulin, without which cells can't take up glucose to use as energy. But fast-acting carbohydrates such as sugar, refined flour, white rice, pasta, and potatoes have a high "glycemic index"—that is, they turn into blood glucose much more quickly than carbohydrates in high-fiber foods such as fruits, vegetables, legumes, and whole grains. The abrupt infusion of blood sugar from fast-acting carbohydrates unleashes a surge of insulin so great

that it overshoots the metabolic mark and drives blood-sugar levels lower than normal. Low blood sugar makes us feel hungry, so we reach for another high-glycemic-index carbohydrate—starting the whole cycle all over again.

David Ludwig, M.D., director of the obesity program at Children's Hospital Boston, and other researchers have begun studying weight-loss diets designed to curb appetite by smoothing out the wild gyrations of blood sugar and insulin that occur on diets of high-glycemic-index carbohydrates. In one study, Ludwig put a group of overweight children on a standard low-fat diet and a comparison group on a low-glycemic diet. The low-glycemic dieters were instructed to combine protein, healthful fat, and low-glycemic carbohydrates like fruits, vegetables, legumes, and whole grains at each meal. After four months, children on the low-glycemic diet had lost an average of 4.5 pounds, while the kids on the low-fat diet had gained 2.9 pounds.

Low-glycemic meals seem to curb hunger in adults, too, according to a recent study of a dozen overweight men by scientists from Laval University in Quebec. On their own, the men consumed 25 percent fewer calories on a low-glycemic diet than on a standard low-fat diet. Moreover, their triglyceride levels improved. More than half our five-year successes who tried "eating fewer carbohydrates like bread and potatoes" also said it helped them lose weight and keep it off.

2. Don't skimp on protein.

Traditional reducing diets restrict protein intake to 15 percent of calories. Yet according to Gary Foster, Ph.D., clinical director of the weight- and eating-disorders program at the University of Pennsylvania School of Medicine in Philadelphia, "If you add protein to the diet, it basically slows the absorption of food." If you eat a platter of fish with some white rice, for example, your blood sugar will rise more slowly than if you consume the same number of calories as rice alone—making protein a useful part of a low-glycemic diet.

Ludwig, of Children's Hospital Boston, demonstrated the hunger-curbing power of a higher-protein diet with an ingenious experiment involving a dozen overweight teenage boys. On one test day, they ate a high-glycemic breakfast and lunch containing lots of easily digested carbohydrates but very little fat and protein. On another day,

Are you getting enough fiber?

Most Americans don't eat enough fiber, according to the new fiber-intake guidelines from the National Academies' Institute of Medicine, which formulates dietary recommendations for the government. The average American adult consumes only 14 to 15 grams of fiber per day. The IOM standard, set in September 2002, suggests 25 grams a day for women, 38 grams a day for men ages 19 to 50, and 21 and 30 grams, respectively, for women and men over age 50. Those levels are slightly higher than the 20 to 35 grams of daily fiber long advocated by the National Cancer Institute and other health organizations.

In addition to its proven benefits for heart disease—on which the IOM recommendations are based—fiber plays a role in weight loss, diabetes management, and relief of constipation. For decades, research suggested that fiber also helps protect against colon cancer, in part by speeding potentially cancer-causing wastes through the colon. While conflicting findings over the last several years brought that benefit into question, the two most recent large observational studies found that people who eat diets high in fiber indeed have a significantly lower risk of developing precancerous polyps or the cancer itself, compared with those who eat little fiber.

AN APPLE A DAY...

To meet the fiber standard, aim to eat several servings of whole grains and five to nine servings of fruits and vegetables daily, plus regular doses of legumes (beans, lentils, split peas) and other fiber-rich foods such as nuts and seeds. Finding whole-grain breads or cereals requires some vigilance, since some labeled "multigrain" or "wheat" may contain little or no fiber. Look for products that list a whole grain—such as whole wheat, whole or rolled oats, kamut, or barley—as their first ingredient. Breads should have at least 2 grams of fiber per slice.

Eating more fiber doesn't have to mean drastically altering your eating habits; focus instead on making small changes over time. Start by substituting just a few servings of fiber-rich foods for lower-fiber ones: Choose whole-grain cereal or oatmeal in place of refined-grain cereal, or a quesadilla with beans and vegetables instead of plain cheese. Then continue increasing your fiber intake gradually over several weeks. Don't rush, since eating too much fiber too soon can cause gas, bloating, and other digestive distress. And don't overdo it: Excessive intake can hamper the absorption of certain minerals, notably calcium, iron, and zinc, and huge amounts of fiber can cause intestinal blockage.

You don't have to worry about what "type" of fiber each food contains. Foods higher in soluble fiber (oats and most fruits) have historically been promoted for lowering cholesterol, while those higher in insoluble fiber (whole grains and most vegetables) have been touted for their gastrointestinal benefits. But that distinction is becoming less relevant as researchers discover significant overlap in the health benefits of soluble and insoluble fiber-rich foods.

While fiber supplements may be appropriate for some people, such as those who suffer from constipation, it's generally best to get your fiber from foods, not pills. Most fiber-rich foods also provide a range of other beneficial vitamins, minerals, and other nutrients. And the evidence for the benefits of high-fiber foods is much stronger than that for fiber alone.

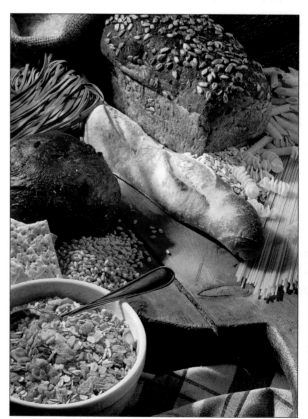

Whole-grain foods are a rich source of fiber, which plays a major role in a healthy diet.

they ate a low-glycemic breakfast and lunch that contained about twice as much protein and 50 percent more fat but only two-thirds as much carbohydrates as the high-glycemic meals. The calorie content of both meals was identical. After consuming their test breakfasts and lunches, the boys were allowed to eat as much dinner as they wanted from platters laden with bagels, cold cuts, cream cheese, cookies, and fruit. On the days when they'd previously eaten high-glycemic meals, the boys scarfed down 81 percent more calories at dinner than on the days when they'd eaten the high-protein, low-glycemic meals.

A bowl of chicken soup will fill you up faster than the same amount of chicken and noodles served on a plate.

We didn't get food diaries from our dieters, which might have shown whether the weight-loss regimens offered in best-selling books were truly effective. Nonetheless, our dieters said they found several authors helpful in losing and keeping off weight. Among them were Bill Phillips (*Body for Life*); Robert C. Atkins, M.D. (*Dr. Atkins' New Diet Revolution*); and H. Leighton Steward (*SugarBusters!*). Although we have not evaluated the authors' diets, we know they all advocate protein as a mainstay of low-glycemic weight-loss plans.

Nancy Vascellaro, a New York City special-education coordinator with years of failed diets behind her, lost 30 pounds four years ago after she took the advice of a nutritionist and ate protein at practically every meal and snack, while cutting her consumption of high-glycemic carbohydrates by more than half. "It's been very doable because

A plan of your own

To slim down, you don't need Weight Watchers, Jenny Craig, Slim Fast, herbal supplements, or prescription drugs. You can fashion your own weight-loss (and maintenance) program by following these guidelines:

• Consume fewer calories than you burn. A 40-year-old, 6-foot-tall man weighing 225 pounds uses about 2,832 calories a day without physical activity. A woman, age 40, 5 feet, 6 inches tall and weighing 175 pounds, burns about 2,061 calories.

• Choose lean protein such as reduced-fat dairy products, egg whites, fish, chicken, and lean cuts of beef and pork.

• Minimize your consumption of quickly digested carbohydrates such as white rice, sugar, pasta, refined grains, and potatoes as well as products containing corn syrup.

• Whenever you eat such carbohydrates, keep portions small and combine them with protein.

• Eat generous quantities of watery foods such as fruits and vegetables.

• Try to develop a taste for high-fiber grains and legumes such as oatmeal, brown rice, whole-wheat bread, lentils, and chickpeas.

• Include in your diet small quantities of healthful fats such as olive oil, avocados, nuts, olives, and fatty fish (like salmon).

• Do whatever it takes to fit exercise into your life. Take the stairs instead of the elevator. Go on a walk at lunchtime. Park your car a block away from your destination.

• Try to make some form of weight and resistance training a part of your exercise routine.

Chickpeas, black beans, lentils, and other fiber-rich legumes are also good sources of protein.

I've never been hungry," Vascellaro says. "If I want extra food for dinner, instead of having an extra portion of pasta, I'll reach for an extra piece of chicken."

3. Avoid dense foods.
A distended stomach is one signal of satiety with which we're all familiar. Scientists are now learning that dieters can trick their stomachs into feeling that way by choosing foods that have relatively few calories per unit of volume. The idea is that you'll feel full before you've consumed too many calories.

Barbara Rolls and her Penn State colleagues demonstrated the density proposition in an elaborate experiment in which volunteers were offered a series of entrées—a cheese-and-egg casserole, a taco salad, and a baked-pasta dish—each painstakingly formulated in three versions of varying density to be similar in taste and volume, except that the low-density versions had 35 to 40 percent fewer calories than the high-density ones. Allowed to eat as much as they wanted, the volunteers consumed virtually identical volumes of the entrées. When the experiment was over, the volunteers had eaten 20 percent fewer calories of the low-density meals than of the high-density ones.

The easiest way to lower the energy density of food is to add water and fiber and to reduce fat. A bowl of chicken-noodle soup, for instance, will fill you up faster than the same amount of chicken and noodles served side by side on a plate. Interestingly, Rolls' experiments show that just drinking water on the side doesn't contribute to satiety; the water has to be part of the food.

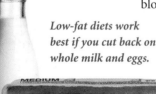
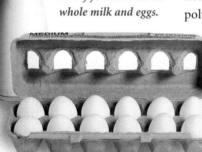

Low-fat diets work best if you cut back on whole milk and eggs.

The foods with the lowest energy density—water-rich fruits and vegetables, whole grains, and lean meats—are the same foods that lower the glycemic index. And whether or not they were aware of the theory behind it, our successful pound-shedders appear to have used energy density to their advantage. About 70 percent of those who tried said that eating fruits, vegetables, and lower-fat foods had helped them lose weight and keep it off.

The "good" fats in nuts may help reduce the risk of heart disease.

4. Have a little fat.
The standard prescription for weight loss is to reduce fat to 30 percent or less of total calories. The National Institutes of Health and the American Heart Association both endorse a low-fat diet as a proven means of preventing heart disease.

Diet surveys show that Americans have heeded the "fat is bad" message by cutting back on foods like whole milk, red meat, and eggs in the last 10 years or so. But, says Kathy McManus, R.D., director of the nutrition department at Boston's Brigham and Women's Hospital, "What the American public chose to eat instead of fat was not zucchini, asparagus, and kidney beans, but refined carbohydrates such as fat-free frozen yogurt, fat-free cookies, pretzels, rice cakes, and graham crackers."

Some obesity researchers are now reconsidering their anti-fat hard line. Recent research shows that replacing fat with high-glycemic carbohydrates can wreak havoc on blood-triglyceride levels even if it helps shed weight. Also, long-term studies have shown that eating certain healthful kinds of fats—notably, mono- and poly-unsaturated vegetable oils, nuts, and fish oil—seems to protect people against heart disease. Most important, however, is new evidence that allowing people to eat a bit more fat than previously permitted can motivate them to stay on their weight-loss plan long enough to show measurable results—and maintain them.

In a clinical trial reported in October 2001, McManus and her colleagues divided 101 overweight men and women into two groups. One followed a standard low-calorie, high-carbohydrate diet restricting fat to 20 percent of calories. The other group followed a diet equally low in total calories with as much as 35 percent of those calories coming from sources of healthful fats such as nuts, fish, and olive oil.

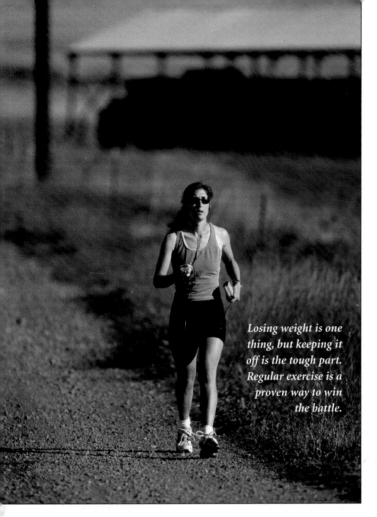

Losing weight is one thing, but keeping it off is the tough part. Regular exercise is a proven way to win the battle.

5. Keep at it. The supersuccessful and unsuccessful dieters used similar weight-loss strategies. They reduced portion sizes, ate more fruits and veggies, cut back on fat, and avoided sweets and junk food. So why did some succeed while others failed? Persistence. More than half of the supersuccesses said they applied those strategies to their diets every day, and another 30 percent did so a few times a week. By contrast, only 20 percent of the failures used the strategies every day, and 35 percent a few times a week.

"Regardless of what people do for dieting and exercise, the longer they do it, the more successful they are," says Robert Jeffery, Ph.D., a professor of epidemiology at the University of Minnesota. "It's not what people do, it's how consistent they are about it. You don't have to be 100 percent, but you have to be better than 10 percent."

MAINTAINING THE LOSS

While it seems that successful dieters can take many paths to reach that longed-for ideal—or at least lower—weight, most used the same tactic to stay there: exercise. Indeed, regular exercise was the No. 1 successful weight-loss maintenance strategy, cited by 81 percent of the long-term maintainers who tried it. Sixty-three percent of five-year maintainers exercised at least three days a week, compared with only 29 percent of those who failed to lose any weight at all. In second place, at 74 percent, was the related strategy of increasing physical activity in daily routines—using stairs instead of the elevator, for example.

Our results track closely with those of the National Weight Control Registry, a database of more than 3,000 people who've lost at least 30 pounds and kept it off for at least a year. (To sign up, call 800-606-6927 or visit its Web site at *www.nwcr.ws.*)

The study lasted for the unusually long period of 18 months. At first, the two groups were losing weight at about the same rate; but as the study wore on, members of the moderate-fat group began to pull ahead. About 60 percent of each group came back for a final weigh-in. The results were telling: People in the low-fat group had gained an average of 6.4 pounds, while the moderate-fat group had lost an average of 9 pounds.

The moderate-fat group also developed healthier eating habits. They added an extra serving of vegetables a day compared with when they started, while the low-fat dieters were eating one serving less. It makes sense that people would boost intake of vegetables made more palatable with a little fat. After all, says McManus, "How much steamed broccoli can you stand over time? It's nice to cook it with a little bit of garlic and olive oil."

Exercise not only burns calories but may help reduce your hunger.

Just 9 percent of the registry members maintain their weight without exercise; about 17 percent of our long-term maintainers said they did not exercise.

Both in our survey and in the registry's data, walking is by far the most common form of exercise. Both of our successful groups—those who lost 10 percent of their weight and kept it off for a year and our superlosers who maintained for five years—did much more weight lifting than the population at large, however. In our sample of superlosers, a full 30 percent said they lifted weights, while only 14 percent of failures did so. The few studies of weight lifting's effectiveness in maintaining weight loss have been inconclusive. But the idea makes physiological sense: Ounce for ounce, muscle tissue is metabolically more active than fat and therefore burns more calories.

Successful weight-loss maintainers in the registry were indefatigable exercisers; their average weekly calorie expenditure was the equivalent of an hour of brisk walking per day. James Hill, of the University of Colorado and codirector of the registry, believes that long-term maintenance of weight loss is all but impossible without rigorous exercise. "Exercise itself may act to regulate hunger" over and above the fact that it burns up calories, Hill says.

The vital role of exercise, however, applies more to the maintenance of weight loss than to losing weight in the first place. A 1999 analysis of the effectiveness of exercise for weight loss, at Brown University School of Medicine in Providence, R.I., showed that while exercise is beneficial, the effects are often modest. There is no escaping the evidence: To take pounds off, change your eating patterns.

Diet and exercise work for kids, too

Children, like their parents, are putting on the pounds. Government health statistics show that 15 percent of all kids between ages 6 and 19 are overweight—up from 4 to 6 percent in the early 1970s. And overweight kids, like overweight adults, can face serious health problems.

A study published in 2003 in the American Heart Association's journal *Circulation* includes a sobering finding: The arteries of overweight children act very much like those of middle-aged smokers. Prof. Kam S. Woo, M.D., of the Department of Medicine and Therapeutics at Prince of Wales Hospital at the Chinese University of Hong Kong and the study's principal author, says: "This carries great health implications and should prompt parents and public-health authorities to do more to deal with the effects of overweight and obesity in children."

Prof. Woo and his colleagues enlisted 82 overweight children ages 9 to 12 to study the effects of diet, exercise, or both on their arteries. Half the kids observed a low-fat, moderate-calorie diet; the others followed the diet and a twice-weekly exercise regimen. The initial test lasted six weeks; afterward the diet-only group and half the diet-and-exercise group kept at it, but with exercise reduced to a weekly session. The researchers checked the kids' body-mass index (a standard measure of obesity), cholesterol levels, and the size and condition of their arteries.

At the end of six weeks, the researchers saw little change in weight or body-mass index, but significant reductions in the so-called "bad" cholesterol levels and significant improvements in the conditions of their arteries. The diet-plus-exercise group showed the greatest improvement.

At the end of a year, the kids who continued the diet-and-exercise regimen continued to show significant improvements in cholesterol levels and the health of their arteries.

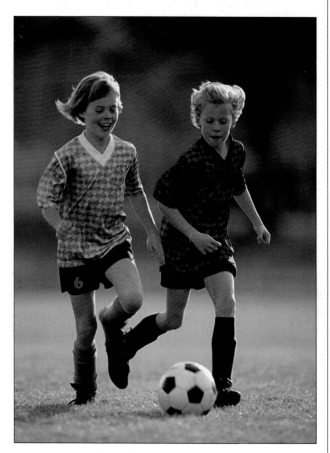

Beyond eating well, young children should exercise regularly, too.

Exotic fruits and vegetables to enhance your diet

Today a typical grocery store carries about 430 different fresh fruits and vegetables—nearly two and a half times the number available in 1980. Thanks to a boom in imports and new, domestic versions of hot sellers, once rare exotic and specialty fruits and vegetables have become commonplace in American markets.

However, with nearly three out of four Americans not meeting the minimum five-a-day standard for fruits and vegetables, too few people are taking advantage of the available variety. To encourage you to expand your dietary repertoire, we've included descriptions, preparation instructions, and nutrition information for some flavorful, nutritious items that have yet to find their way to many American tables. Note that in the descriptions for each entry, an excellent source of a nutrient per serving contains 25 percent or more of the Daily Value of that nutrient; a very good source contains 15 to 24 percent, and a good source contains 5 to 14 percent of the Daily Value.

TASTE AND HEALTH BENEFITS

Eating a variety of produce has an enormous health payoff. Reams of evidence link produce to a reduced risk of deadly or disabling disease, including the big three killers: cancer, heart attack, and stroke. Produce of different colors contains different phytochemicals, or disease-fighting substances. Unusual fruits and vegetables can make it easier to eat a colorful diet that includes red, white, blue, yellow, and green produce.

Fruits and vegetables also contain plenty of fiber, which makes you feel fuller longer (leaving less room for unhealthy foods) and is a disease-fighter in its own right. A pooling of data from 10 epidemiological studies, involving nearly 350,000 adults, found a significant trend toward reduced heart disease with increasing fiber intake, especially from fruit. Every additional 10 grams of fruit fiber that people consumed per day reduced their risk of dying of a cardiac event by 30 percent, according to the February 2004 study in the *Archives of Internal Medicine.*

If you're not feeling adventurous enough for, say, a horned melon, you can start with different varieties of a fruit or vegetable you already know. Blood oranges, for example, are less acidic than regular oranges and make an attractive

red juice. Blue potatoes have a creamy texture and nutty flavor that's perfect for baking. Red bananas are small, dense, and sweet, making them ideal for a fruit tray or lunchbox dessert. Even the more unusual items are often staples in other countries and are simple to prepare.

SAFE PREPARATION OF PRODUCE

The only caveat about eating fresh produce is that you must wash it thoroughly first. Food-borne illness from produce is on the rise as imports from around the globe, with complicated distribution channels, provide many opportunities for contamination. For produce that won't be peeled, rinse or scrub under running water. Even produce that will be peeled or eaten off the rind should be washed with either a produce wash (available in supermarkets) or well-diluted soap and water and rinsed to avoid transferring contaminants from your hands or the knife to the edible parts. Wash items just before you prepare them, not before storage, as it can hasten spoiling.

FRUITS

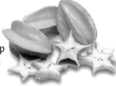

Carambola/Star Fruit
Star-shaped cross sections have a juicy, crisp flesh that combines apple, grape, and citrus flavors. Thin, waxy skin is edible.

- **Look for:** Firm, full fruit with juicy-looking ribs. When ripe, fruit turns yellow and emits a fruity, floral fragrance.
- **To prepare:** Slice horizontally into star shapes and remove any seeds. Eat fresh, slice into fruit salads, or use to garnish seafood, poultry, and drinks. Makes a showy upside-down cake.
- **Nutrients:** Excellent source of vitamin C. Very good source of fiber. Good source of vitamin B6, folate, potassium, and copper.

Cherimoya/Custard Apple
Creamy flesh tastes like a mixture of pineapple, mango, and strawberry.

- **Look for:** A dark-green-colored fruit that yields to gentle pressure. Avoid fruits that are soft or splotched with dark areas. If fruit is still hard and unripe, allow it to soften slightly at room temperature.
- **To prepare:** Serve chilled. Halve or slice into wedges and spoon out fruit, discarding seeds.
- **Nutrients:** Excellent source of vitamin B6, vitamin C, and fiber. Very good source of potassium, riboflavin, and thiamin. Good source of copper, folate, pantothenic acid, magnesium, and phosphorus.

Kiwano/Horned Melon

Bright green gel-like flesh combines the tastes of watermelon, cucumber, and bananas.

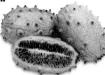

• **Look for:** Bright orange shell with no bruises or spots.
• **To prepare:** Cut in half and scoop out the flesh. Seeds are numerous but edible. Eat as is with a sprinkle of sugar or use in fruit salads or as a garnish with roasted meats. The shell makes a striking container for soups or salads.
• **Nutrients:** Excellent source of vitamin C. Good source of vitamin A and iron.

Kumquat

Olive-sized citrus fruit with a juicy, sweet rind and tart flesh.

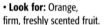

• **Look for:** Orange, firm, freshly scented fruit.
• **To prepare:** Eat out of hand or slice and serve in salads. Try blanching the fruit in boiling water for 20 seconds, dunk in ice water, dry, and slice thinly. Add the slices to salads made from meat, fish, fruits, and vegetables.
• **Nutrients:** Good source of fiber and vitamin C.

Passion Fruit

Dark plum-colored, wrinkled globe encases jellylike golden flesh with a sweet-tart flavor and edible soft seeds.

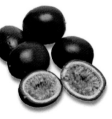

• **Look for:** Fragrant, wrinkled, shriveled fruit that is richly colored. If skin is smooth, ripen at room temperature, turning occasionally.
• **To prepare:** Halve fruit and scoop out the pulp and seeds with a spoon. Eat as is, spoon over fruit and ice cream, or strain and use the juice in drinks and recipes.
• **Nutrients:** Good source of fiber and vitamins A and C.

Tomatillo

This small, green member of the tomato family typically comes encased in a husk and has a sweet-sour flavor used in salsa verde and other Southwest dishes.

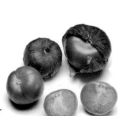

• **Look for:** Firm fruit with a dry, close-fitting husk that shows no blackness or mold.
• **To prepare:** Peel off the husk and wash. Roast or poach for a few minutes to soften the firm skin. Typically diced and cooked into sauces.
• **Nutrients:** Good source of vitamin C.

Ugli Fruit/Uniq Fruit

Large, easily peeled citrus fruit. Yellow-orange sections have few seeds and taste like a combination of grapefruit and mandarin orange.

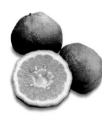

• **Look for:** Fruit that is lime green to bright yellow or orange and fragrant. The thick skin may be unevenly colored and scarred.
• **To prepare:** Peel and section or halve like a grapefruit.
• **Nutrients:** Excellent source of vitamin C. Good source of calcium, fiber, folate, potassium, thiamin, and vitamin A.

VEGETABLES

Asparation/Broccolini

A cross between broccoli and kale, it tastes like tender, sweet broccoli with a bit of an asparagus bite.

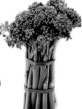

• **Look for:** Crisp stalks with green (not yellow) heads.
• **To prepare:** Steam, sauté, or stir-fry until tender-crisp. Use like broccoli or asparagus in recipes.
• **Nutrients:** Excellent source of vitamins A and C. Good source of calcium, fiber, and potassium.

Baby Bok Choy

Miniature version of bok choy, which has a taste similar to Swiss chard or spinach. Cooking enhances the flavor, making it milder and sweeter.

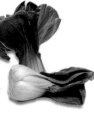

• **Look for:** Heads with full green leaves, white stalks.
• **To prepare:** Rinse, shake dry, and drain thoroughly. Leave whole or slice stalks crosswise and sauté, stir-fry, or add to soups. When preparing larger bok choy, separate the stalks from the leaves, as they take longer to cook.
• **Nutrients:** Very good source of vitamin A. Good source of calcium.

Chayote

Versatile, squash-like vegetable with a pale, crisp flesh that combines the flavors of cucumber and zucchini.

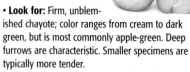

• **Look for:** Firm, unblemished chayote; color ranges from cream to dark green, but is most commonly apple-green. Deep furrows are characteristic. Smaller specimens are typically more tender.
• **To prepare:** Peel with a vegetable peeler before cooking, or afterward by pulling off the skin. Then use as you would any summer squash—pureed, steamed, sautéed, sliced in salads, or baked. The firm texture holds up better than many squashes when stuffed or sliced. The seeds are edible and can be cooked along with the squash.
• **Nutrients:** Excellent source of folate. Very good source of vitamin C. Good source of copper, fiber, and zinc.

Rainbow Chard

A milder-flavored version of the typical red or green Swiss chard. Stalks have a celerylike flavor and leaves have a beetlike flavor.

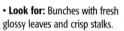

• **Look for:** Bunches with fresh glossy leaves and crisp stalks.
• **To prepare:** Leaves and stalks are often used separately, either raw or cooked. Leaves can be used in salads or substituted for spinach in recipes. Stalks work well in recipes calling for asparagus. Cook lightly to retain the bright colors.
• **Nutrients:** Excellent source of vitamin A. Very good source of vitamin C. Good source of magnesium.

Sunflower Chokes/ Sunchoke/Jerusalem Artichoke

Despite the popular moniker, these lumpy, brown-skinned sunflower roots are not an artichoke and do not come from Jerusalem. The white flesh of these chokes is nutty, crunchy, crisp, and sweet.

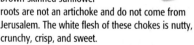

• **Look for:** Chokes that are firm and fresh-looking, not soft or wrinkled.
• **To prepare:** Serve raw with dips or in salads; roast like a potato; or boil, steam, sauté, or stir-fry alone or with other vegetables.
• **Nutrients:** Excellent source of iron. Very good source of thiamin and potassium. Good source of copper, fiber, folate, magnesium, niacin, phosphorus, riboflavin, vitamin B6, and vitamin C.

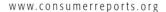

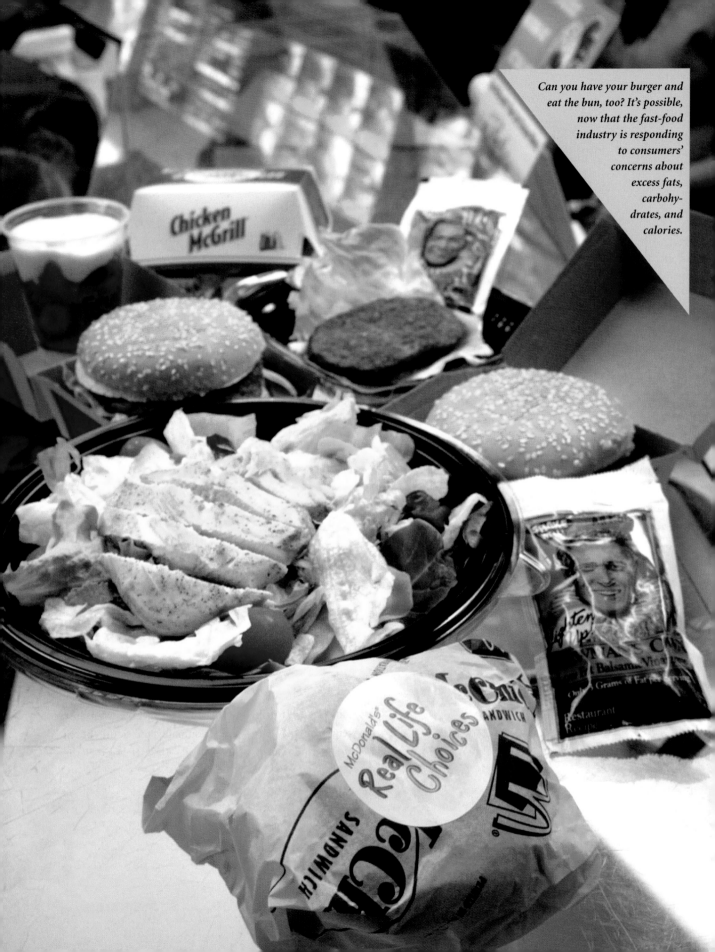

Can you have your burger and eat the bun, too? It's possible, now that the fast-food industry is responding to consumers' concerns about excess fats, carbohydrates, and calories.

The new, healthier *fast food*

With health-conscious consumers seeking lean, nutritious meals when they're on the go, and lawyers warming up the obesity lawsuits, the fast-food industry is feeling the heat. The major chains are increasingly trying to offer healthy options, from bunless burgers for the low-carb Atkins crowd to grilled chicken and salads for the fat-and-calorie counters.

Most of the new items are a boon to consumers wanting to eat cheap, fast, and healthy. Fast-food restaurants today "pretty much all have something on the menu that's designed to be a healthier choice," says Marion Nestle, Ph.D., department chair for nutrition, food studies, and public health at New York University. But you need to know how to separate the healthy from the hype. For example, Burger King's low-carbohydrate, bunless Double-Meat Whopper With Cheese contains a whopping 630 calories and 47 grams of total fat.

Here's how to cobble together reasonably lean, nutritious meals when you're grazing in the junk-food jungle.

THE LOW-CARB CRAZE

The fast-food industry has started responding to the unprecedented success of the Atkins, South Beach, and other low-carbohydrate diets by making certain simple changes. Most notably, restaurants are offering burgers without the bun (served on a plate at Burger King or wrapped in a lettuce leaf at Hardee's) and letting you substitute other items for French fries and sodas in the bargain meals.

Cutting back on foods such as white-flour buns, soft drinks, and sweets, which contain lots of refined carbohydrates, is a good idea for everyone because they're generally low in nutrients and fiber. Moreover, those foods—as well as potatoes—have a high glycemic index, which means they're digested quickly, causing blood sugar to surge and then plummet a few hours later. That process creates a sensation of hunger and may stimulate overeating. It may also increase the level of triglycerides, a potentially harmful fat in the blood, and decrease the "good" HDL-cholesterol level. That's a particular concern for the estimated one-fourth of Americans who have a prediabetic disorder called the metabolic syndrome.

However, discarding the bun does not provide carte blanche to gorge on burgers and cheeseburgers, which tend to contain lots of calories and artery-clogging saturated fat. Studies show that while the Atkins diet, for example, may help control hunger, people who lose weight on that diet—and presumably the South Beach and other low-carb diets as well—ultimately do it the same way as other dieters: by ingesting fewer total calories. And perhaps in a nod to extensive research linking saturated fat to heart disease and other health problems, even Atkins Nutritionals, the company founded by the late Dr. Atkins, is now saying that the program "does not give you license to stuff yourself with fatty meats and cheese," which are high in saturated fat.

A better choice than burgers is one of the meal-sized salads topped with a low-calorie dressing plus a variety of fruits, vegetables, nuts, and lean meats offered by most of the large chains. (See the accompanying table, "Fast-food sampler.") Or try one of the whole-grain wraps at Subway or the Carb-Counter sandwiches at Blimpie—both made with low-carb, low-glycemic breads. But hold the bacon and substitute a low-fat dressing. Or customize a sandwich using those breads, lean meat or chicken, and vegetables. (Try to avoid the wheat rolls at both Blimpie and Subway, which contain mostly enriched white flour.) Any of those choices will give you a low-glycemic meal that's "a good lunch for anyone, not just those watching their weight or blood-sugar level," says Susan Roberts, Ph.D., professor of nutrition at Tufts University in Boston.

In general, the healthier choices listed in the table also contain less sodium than a typical fastfood meal, which can easily exceed the 2,400-milligram maximum that government agencies suggest for an entire day. However, many of those choices are still fairly high in sodium, particularly for individuals who have high blood pressure or a family history of that condition.

More and more fast-food diners are opting not to get fries.

MORE AND BETTER CHOICES

In addition to low-carb offerings, most fast-food restaurants also target products to people who are counting calories and fat. The chains have done that by expanding their menus to include lean meats, fresh produce, and more condiment options. Where it used to be a choice of just mayo or mustard, you can now top your sandwiches with grilled peppers and onions or a fat-free sweet onion sauce.

There's also a trend toward doing away with the "healthy-choice penalty," the extra cost you pay for substituting other items for the fries and soda. At some restaurants you can build a meal with a sandwich, side salad, and choice of low-fat or skim milk, juice, tea, or bottled water and still pay the bargain-meal price.

SMART STRATEGIES

If you eat typical fast-food fare more than occasionally, you could be adversely affecting your overall diet—and your health. A study of 17,000 children and adults published in the October 2003 issue of the *Journal of the American Dietetic Association* found that on days when people ate the usual fast food, they consumed more calories, fat, and sodium and less of the healthful nutrients than they did on other days.

But eating out doesn't have to cause a nutritional shortfall if you follow these smart-eating strategies:

Plan ahead. Fast-food restaurants provide a wealth of nutritional information through the Internet and toll-free numbers as well as brochures available in the restaurants. Many Web sites provide nutritional calculators that let you customize your menu choices and then check the nutritional totals.

Control portion size. Supersizing your burger, fries, and soda may seem like a bargain, but doing so can cost you up to 1,000 extra calories.

Focus on vegetables, fruits, and whole grains. Go for large salads or, if you want a sandwich, choose whole-grain breads, double the vegetable toppings, and substitute a salad for the accompanying chips or fries.

Shun fried foods. A fried chicken breast, for example, has 80 percent more calories than a broiled breast and five times the saturated fat.

Try a different topping. Most restaurants offer flavorful alternatives to high-fat, high-calorie condiments such as butter, mayonnaise, sour cream, and bacon. At Subway, for example, you can choose from six different fat-free dressings and sandwich spreads. If you must have a high-fat dressing, try this trick: Pour the dressing on the side and dip the tines of your fork in it before each bite.

Count your drink and dessert. Reach for diet soda, tea, or bottled water instead of sugared sodas or high-fat shakes, which can more than double a meal's calories. Low-fat or skim milk provides calcium, protein, and vitamins D and B12. (So does cheese, but it has more fat and calories.) The best dessert choices—low-fat yogurt and ice cream—are also good sources of calcium.

Fast-food sampler

Traditional fast-food items listed first, followed by healthier alternatives.

Food	Serving (ounces)	Calories	Total fat (grams)	Saturated fat (grams)	Sodium (milligrams)
BURGER KING					
Whopper with cheese	11.1	800	50	18	1,420
Santa Fe Fire-Grilled Chicken Baguette	7.6	350	5	1.5	1,220
BK Veggie Burger with reduced-fat mayo	6.1	300	7	1	870
Fire-Grilled Caesar Chicken Salad (no garlic toast)					
• Caesar dressing	12.5	330	17.5	5	1,540
• Fat-Free Ranch dressing	12.0	290	7	3	1,470
McDONALD'S					
Quarter Pounder with cheese	7.0	540	29	13	1,240
Chicken McGrill without mayo	7.0	300	7	4.5	940
Grilled Chicken Cobb salad					
• Cobb dressing	12.7	390	20	6.5	1,500
• Low-fat balsamic vinaigrette	12.2	310	14	5	1,790
Fruit 'n Yogurt Parfait	5.3	160	2	1	85
Vanilla Reduced-Fat Ice-Cream Cone	3.2	150	4.5	3	75
WENDY'S					
Big Bacon Classic Hamburger	9.9	580	29	12	1,430
Mandarin Chicken Salad with almonds					
• Oriental sesame dressing	15.3	570	33	4.5	1,370
• Fat-Free French dressing	15.3	400	14	2	1,020
Classic Single Hamburger without mayo	7.4	380	16	6	855
Baked potato with broccoli and cheese (no butter)	14.0	340	3	1	430
Grilled Chicken Sandwich with honey-mustard sauce	6.6	300	6	1.5	730
BLIMPIE					
Ultimate BLT Wrap	10.0	831	50	15	2,677
Seafood Sub	11.0	355	7.7	1.6	895
Tuscan Ham and Swiss (Carb-Counter menu)	10.4	340	13	6	1,450
SUBWAY					
Foot-long Meatball Sub	20.2	1,080	52	22	2,580
Chicken Ranch Wrap with Fat-Free Ranch (no bacon)	8.3	325	8.5	3	1,465
6-inch Turkey Breast and Ham Sub	8.1	290	5	1.5	1,220
PIZZA HUT					
1 slice large Stuffed Crust Supreme Pizza	6.2	400	16	8	1,070
1 slice large Fit 'N Delicious* Pizza with ham, onion, and mushroom	3.3	150	4	2	440
TACO BELL					
Grilled Stuffed Beef Burrito	11.4	730	33	11	2,080
Steak Burrito Supreme "Fresco Style"	8.5	350	9	2.5	1,260
Chicken Soft Taco "Fresco Style"**	4.0	170	4	1	560

Chart originally appeared in the April 2004 issue of CONSUMER REPORTS.
The FDA's recommended daily maximums for adults, based on a 2,000-calorie diet, are: total fat, 65 grams; saturated fat, 20 grams; fiber, 25 grams; sodium, 2,400 milligrams.
* Fit 'N Delicious pizza is made with thin crust and half the usual amount of cheese.
** "Fresco Style" substitutes a chunky salsa for sauce and cheese.

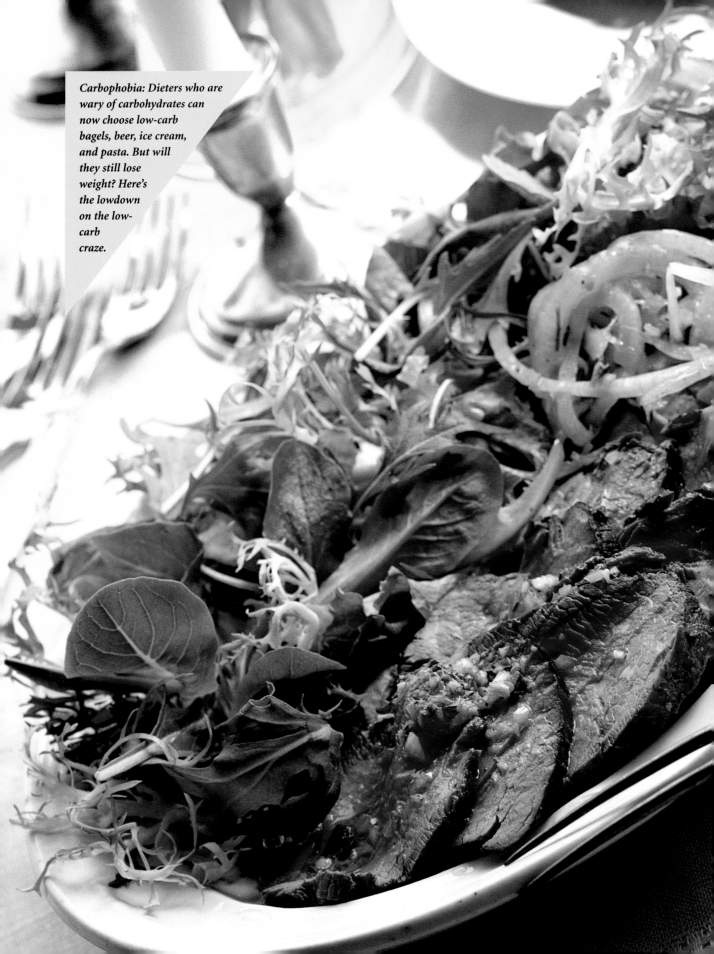

Carbophobia: Dieters who are wary of carbohydrates can now choose low-carb bagels, beer, ice cream, and pasta. But will they still lose weight? Here's the lowdown on the low-carb craze.

The skinny on low-carb foods

When is a calorie not a calorie? When it comes from a low-carbohydrate food. That, at least, is what many food advertisements and labels now imply.

"For just 3 grams of net carbs per serving, you can reward yourself with one of life's most delicious indulgences," says the label of Keto's low-carb Rt. 66 Rocky Road ice cream. "Only tastes like cheating," says an ad for Carborite's "extraordinarily delicious low carb" cookies and candies.

But a CONSUMER REPORTS investigation has found that many of the low-carb food products now flooding supermarkets may in fact be cheating—consumers, that is—by undermining the weight loss they hope to achieve. Among our findings:

• Using scientifically suspect assumptions, many manufacturers are prominently listing "net carbs" along with the true carbohydrate counts found on products' Nutrition Facts labels.

• "Net carbs" claims are questionable for low-carb versions of comfort foods such as bread, pasta, and ice cream, since they are extrapolated from research done on whole foods with very different composition and calorie content.

• The original low-carb diets probably worked because they were monotonous and low in calories. Today's low-carb comfort foods are neither. A 1-ounce Carborite chocolate crisp bar contains 120 calories. A serving of Keto's Rocky Road has 270 calories, almost double the calories found in many regular ice creams, and twice as much fat.

"If low-carb food is high in calories, we're going to get fat on it," said Joanne Slavin, Ph.D., professor of food science and nutrition at the University of Minnesota. That's why consumers need to know the truth about low-carb labeling and how to ensure that the proliferation of low-carb products doesn't defeat the very diet principles—proven or not—that have made low-carb diets a runaway hit.

If low-carb food is high in calories, we're going to get fat on it.

TRUTH: "Low-carb" labels are meaningless.

An astonishing 930 low-carbohydrate food products were introduced to U.S. markets from 1999-2004. They're aimed at the 16 percent of American adults (an estimated 30 million to 40 million people) who say they're trying to control their weight by counting carbs, not calories, according to a February 2004 Roper Reports survey.

At the same time, the restaurant industry, which has long resisted calls to include calorie counts on menus, seems to have little reluctance to create "low-carb" menu items.

"Rarely does the opportunity to improve the health of the nation collide with a strong potential for profits in the food and beverage industry," wrote Gil Wilshire, M.D.,

Low-carb lingo

To turn high-carbohydrate foods into low-carb versions, food processors are making new uses of old ingredients such as sugar alcohols and fermentable carbohydrates. These substances don't have serious safety issues, though they may produce diarrhea and gas in susceptible people. There's some evidence that they can help with blood-sugar control, but there's no evidence that focusing on foods with these ingredients will help you lose weight.

Net carbohydrates. In most low-carb labeling, "net carbs"

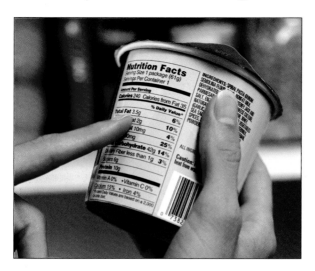

refers to the total grams of carbohydrates per serving minus grams of fiber and sugar alcohols. The term has no legal standing, though the Food and Drug Administration has announced plans to address it and other low-carb claims in regulations.

Sugar alcohols, or polyols (erythritol, hydrogenated starch hydrolysates [HSH], isomalt, lactitol, maltitol, mannitol, sorbitol, xylitol).

Polyols are not digested in the small intestine the way regular sugars are. Instead, they pass through to the large intestine, where they are digested by fermentation. Thus they do not elevate blood sugar and insulin levels nearly as much as regular sugar does, giving them a low glycemic index. But like sugars, which have 4 calories per gram, they do contribute calories, ranging from a low of 0.2 per gram for erythritol to 3 per gram for HSH.

Fermentable carbohydrates (inulin, resistant starch, polydextrose). This catchall refers to smooth, bland-tasting, highly processed ingredients (usually derived from corn) that can be used in place of high-carb white flour and counted as fiber. Fermentable carbohydrates are digested the way sugar alcohols are. They have between 1.6 and 2.5 calories per gram (compared with 4 per gram for regular starches).

---

president of the low-carb trade association, the Carbohydrate Awareness Council, in the February 2004 *Food Product Design*, a trade publication.

Through the miracle of modern food technology, manufacturers have turned high-carb snacks into low-carb products by replacing sugars with sugar alcohols and refined grains with isolated fibers, and resistant starches. Since these ingredients, though technically carbohydrates, move through the small intestine without being absorbed, the Atkins and other product lines subtract them from the total carb count. Hence the term "net carbs" that you see on many labels. (For more on the new lingo, see "Low-carb lingo," above.)

The surge of low-carbohydrate products has been so swift that regulatory agencies are scrambling to catch up. As of now, there's not even an agreed-upon definition of "low-carbohydrate," let alone "net carbs." The Food and

Drug Administration is addressing this issue, but final regulations are probably about a year away. In April 2004, the Department of the Treasury Alcohol and Tobacco Tax and Trade Bureau ruled that labels on wine, beer, and distilled beverages can make statements about total carb counts but not calculate "net carbs" nor imply that these beverages play a healthful role in weight maintenance or reduction.

TRUTH: Not all low-carb foods are equal.

The main principle behind low-carbohydrate diets is that because they steady blood-sugar levels, which spike and then fall dramatically after the consumption of high-carb foods, they decrease appetite and allow dieters to eat more reasonably. Scientific evidence supports that theory. Foods that produce a slow rise in blood sugar—such as high-fiber grains, vegetables, and protein—are said to have a low glycemic index. Fat has a glycemic index of zero because it does not affect blood sugar at all. A growing body of research suggests that diets heavy in low-glycemic foods not only improve cardiovascular risk factors such as cholesterol but also help with weight control because they help people feel fuller longer.

Promoters of low-carb comfort foods say that those foods, too, should be considered low-glycemic products because their sugar alcohols and resistant starches, unlike sugar and regular starches, don't promote a rise in blood sugar. But David Ludwig, M.D., Ph.D., director of the obesity program at Children's Hospital Boston and an authority on low-glycemic diets, notes: "It's one thing to be looking at the glycemic index as one of several factors that influences appetite for natural foods. It's another to create highly processed products, using these compounds which are present at unnaturally high concentrations, and then assuming that those principles that we observed with real foods will continue to apply. It's an example of how commercial claims have vastly outstripped the science."

TRUTH: Low-carb then is not low-carb now.

Ironically, the current flood of low-carb products on the market may make it harder to lose weight on a low-carb diet. In its original form, the Atkins diet severely restricted the carbohydrate-laden foods that on average make up about 50 percent of Americans' calorie intake: bread, pasta, rice, sweetened soft drinks, potato chips, cookies, and even fruits. Dieters were allowed large helpings of the high-fat steaks, cheese, butter, and oils that previous low-fat regimens had denied them. In addition, they could eat large bowls of greens and smaller quantities of other vegetables whose carbohydrate content was sufficiently

Opt for "good" complex carbs, such as breads made from whole grains.

negligible. The chief Atkins competitor, the South Beach Diet, also restricted starchy carbs, fruits, and sugars, but in addition warned dieters away from high-fat meats and dairy foods.

When independent researchers finally got around to studying the Atkins diet objectively, they found, against all their expectations, that low-carb dieters lost weight faster than low-fat dieters, at least for the first six months. (There are no independent published studies on the South Beach Diet.)

A yearlong study of the Atkins diet involved 37 participants and was headed by Gary Foster, Ph.D., of the University of Pennsylvania. In the study, those on the Atkins diet had lost an average of 8.4 pounds more than the low-fat dieters at the end of six months; by the end of the year the gap was so narrow as to be statistically insignificant.

A prime reason the low-carb diet worked, some researchers concluded, was it was boring. "At some point we become so tired of any given thing that we eat that it has no continuing hedonic effect on us," said Brian Wansink, Ph.D., who studies food choices as professor of marketing and nutritional science at the University of Illinois at Champaign. "I almost guarantee that everyone would lose weight on an all-pizza or all-chocolate diet."

Conversely, research by Wansink and many others has shown that the more variety in your diet, the more food you'll eat, as everyone who has dined at a lavish buffet can attest. Taking the boredom out of the low-carb diet with low-carb comfort foods, such as ice cream, chips, and beer, could reduce its effectiveness.

"Originally, the Atkins diet was black-and-white," said Alice H. Lichtenstein, D.Sc., professor of nutrition science and policy at Tufts University. "I can have the steak but not the baked potato. Now I can have the steak, but I can also have the low-carb pasta on the side."

> *At some point we become so tired of any given thing that we eat that it has no continuing hedonic effect on us.*

TRUTH: Low-carb junk food is still junk.

Lost in the media celebration of research that showed positive results for the Atkins diet was the fact that low-carb dieters were actually losing weight the old-fashioned way: by taking in fewer calories than they expended.

A six-month study that actually tracked calorie consumption, headed by Frederick F. Samaha, M.D., of the Philadelphia Veterans Affairs Medical Center, found that by the end of the study, the low-carb dieters reported that they had cut an average of 189 more calories a day than the low-fat dieters. That was more than enough to account for the average 8.5 extra pounds they had shed.

Indeed, the very lack of availability of low-carb junk food might have been a boon for low-carb dieters. Remember SnackWells? Those bright-green packages of cookies may have been the downfall of low-fat dieters who believed that calories be damned, they could eat as many Devil's Food Cookie Cakes as they wanted because those 50-calorie cakes contained 0 grams of fat. Today's low-carbohydrate "indulgences" could create a similar trap. Of the low-carb products introduced in the U.S. in the past five years, 58 percent fall into four categories—bakery, confectionery, desserts and ice cream, and snacks—according to the Mintel International Group, a product-tracking firm. Those products can have almost as many calories as snacks they're designed to replace, despite the big "net carbs" number on the packages' front.

A "serving" of four small foil-wrapped Russell Stover Low Carb Pecan Delight chocolates, for instance, contains a mere 3.2 net carbs, but 190 calories. If you were to fulfill a daily 40-gram net-carb quota entirely with these morsels, you'd consume 2,376 calories.

"Atkins worked as well as it did for people because it got them away from cookies and snack foods they really liked," said Slavin at the University of Minnesota. "Now that these products are available, it's going to be just like low-fat—they're going to eat a lot of it."

WHAT YOU CAN DO

Here are ways to avoid the pitfalls of a low-carb diet:

• **Eat whole foods whenever possible.** "A better diet has fruits, vegetables, and whole grains in it, not mannitol," said Slavin. For 40 grams a day of "net carbs," you could eat a half-cup of lentils, a cup of carrots, an orange, and a slice of light seven-grain bread—for a total of 274 calories—plenty of natural fiber, and a host of vitamins and minerals. By contrast, getting those 40 grams from low-carb snack foods might give you 1,440 calories and few other nutrients.

• **Read the calorie count on the Nutrition Facts label.** Many low-carbohydrate snacks are even higher in fat than their regular counterparts, yet fat doesn't register on the "net carbs" count.

• **Treat treats as treats, no matter what the carb count.** You shouldn't eat five low-carb chocolate bars at a sitting any more than you should eat five regular ones.

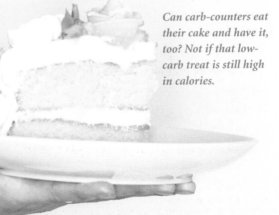

Can carb-counters eat their cake and have it, too? Not if that low-carb treat is still high in calories.

Low-carb food Ratings

Within categories, in order of overall quality.

Product	Serving size	Cost	Calories	Total carbs (g)	Net carbs (g)	Fat (g)
BREAD						
VERY GOOD Slightly sweet with grain flavor and no off-notes; worked very well with toppings.						
Arnold Carb Counting Multi-Grain	1 slice (27 g)	$0.14	60	9	6	2
Sara Lee Delightful Wheat Bakery	1 slice (23 g)	0.10	45	9	7	0
GOOD Grain flavor, but some sour (Atkins) or bitter (Nature's Own) notes. CarbXtract was pleasantly nutty but dry and crumbly; the others were slightly spongy.						
Atkins Bakery Multi-Grain	1 slice (28 g)	0.28	70	7	3	2
CarbXtract Multi-Grain*	1 slice (29 g)	0.41	42	6	5	1
Nature's Own Healthline Wheat'n Fiber	1 slice (28 g)	0.10	60	7	5	1
FAIR Spongy and rubbery, with off-flavors. Toppings might not help.						
Food For Life Low Carbohydrate The Original	1 slice (23 g)	0.22	70	4	3	4
JoeBread Our Original Low Carb	1 slice (21 g)	0.25	49	4	2	2
BAGEL						
GOOD Mildly sweet with a toasted wheat flavor, but texture was more like a soft roll than a bagel.						
Thomas' Carb Counting 100% Whole Wheat	1/2 bagel (31 g)	0.24	70	11	8	1
PASTA						
GOOD Grain flavor, but a bit crumbly, rubbery, and/or dry; pasta sauce may cover those defects.						
Keto Spaghetti	2 oz. dry (56 g)	1.16	197	11	8	2
Bella Vita Low Carb Pasta Penne Rigate	2 oz. dry (56 g)	0.48	160	18	10	1
CarbXtract Fettuccine*	2 oz. dry (56 g)	2.31	168	29	17	2
FAIR Defects such as dry, rubbery, or crumbly texture or starchy taste. Sauce may not help.						
Darielle Pasta Mezze Penne	2 oz. dry (56 g)	0.50	160	18	10	1
Atkins Quick Quisine Spaghetti	2 oz. dry (56 g)	0.92	210	13	5	3
ICE CREAM (vanilla)						
FAIR Gummy, foamy, and/or overly icy, with imitation flavors or artificial-sweetener impressions.						
Goldenbrook Farms LeCarb Frozen Dessert	1/2 cup (63 g)	0.98	100	6	3	7
Atkins Endulge Super Premium Ice Cream	1/2 cup (70 g)	0.91	140	13	3	12
Breyers Carb Smart Ice Cream*	1/2 cup (66 g)	0.33	130	10	4	9
BEER						
GOOD Similar to a light domestic lager, but less intense and with a slight metallic aftertaste. Rolling Rock had a hollow, slightly off-flavor taste and was least impressive.						
Michelob Ultra	12 fl. oz.	0.83	95	3	3	0
Miller Lite	12 fl. oz.	0.71	96	3	3	0
Rolling Rock Rock Green Light	12 fl. oz.	0.69	84	2	2	0

*Products may have been reformulated since our June 2004 test.

GUIDE TO THE RATINGS Ratings are based on flavor and texture quality as judged by trained panelists in blind tests. Ratings for low-carb beers are relative to light beers, not regular domestic lagers. Most products are sold in supermarkets or health-food stores, but CarbXtract Multi-Grain Bread and CarbXtract Fettuccine are not; we purchased those online. **Serving size** and nutrition figures are based on labels, but labeled sizes for Thomas' Carb Counting Bagels, Keto Spaghetti, and CarbXtract Fettuccine were adjusted for comparison. **Cost per serving** is based on approximate retail price. **Net carbs** is based on the labeled "net," or "effective," carbohydrate count; when not labeled, we computed net carbs by subtracting the fiber and sugar-alcohol contents from the total carb count. Note: All nutrition figures are rounded to the nearest whole number. Chart originally appeared in the June 2004 issue of CONSUMER REPORTS.

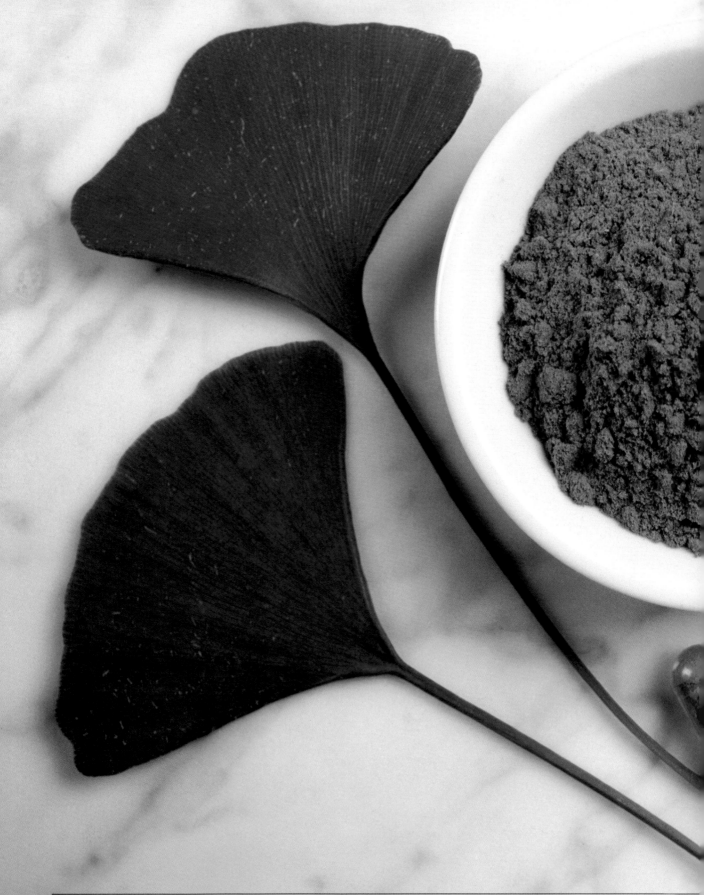

Vitamins & Supplements

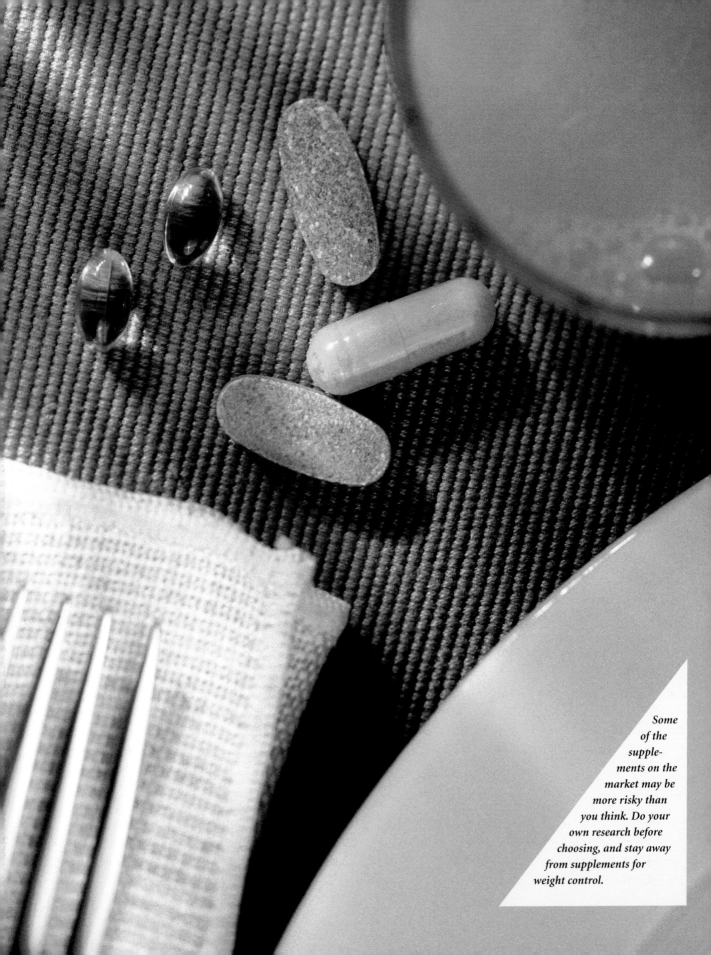

Some of the supplements on the market may be more risky than you think. Do your own research before choosing, and stay away from supplements for weight control.

Dangerous supplements: still at large

If you can buy it at a clean, well-lighted store, if it's "all natural," it's not going to do you serious harm, right? That's what many Americans assume about dietary supplements. But while most supplements are probably fairly benign, CONSUMER REPORTS has identified a dozen that according to government warnings, adverse-event reports, and top experts are too dangerous to be on the market. Yet they are. We easily purchased all 12 in February 2004 in a few days of shopping online and in retail stores.

These unsafe supplements include Aristolochia, an herb conclusively linked to kidney failure and cancer in China, Europe, Japan, and the U.S.; yohimbe, a sexual stimulant linked to heart and respiratory problems; bitter orange, whose ingredients have effects similar to those of the banned weight-loss stimulant ephedra; and chaparral, comfrey, germander, and kava, all known or likely causes of liver failure. (For a complete list of the "dirty dozen," see "Twelve supplements you should avoid," on page 36.)

U.S. consumers shelled out some $76 million in 2002 for just three of these supplements: androstenedione, kava, and yohimbe, the only ones for which sales figures were available, according to the *Nutrition Business Journal*, which tracks the supplement industry.

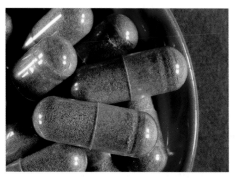

Ephedra capsules like these, aimed at dieters, were recently banned by the FDA.

The potentially dangerous effects of most of these products have been known for more than a decade, and at least five of them are banned in Asia, Europe, or Canada. Yet until very recently, the U.S. Food and Drug Administration had not managed to remove a single dietary supplement from the market for safety reasons.

After seven years of trying, the agency announced a ban on the weight-loss aid ephedra in December 2003. And in March 2004 it warned 23 companies to stop marketing the body-building supplement androstenedione (andro).

Despite these actions against high-profile supplements, whose dangers were so well known that even industry trade groups had stopped defending them, the agency continues to be hamstrung by the 1994 Dietary Supplement Health and Education Act (DSHEA, pronounced de-*shay*). While drug manufacturers are required to prove that their products are safe before being marketed, DSHEA makes the FDA prove that supplements on the market are unsafe and denies the agency all but the sketchiest information about the safety record of most of them.

"The standards for demonstrating a supplement is hazardous are so high that it can take the FDA years to build a case," said Bruce Silverglade, legal director of the Center for Science in the Public Interest, a Washington, D.C., consumer-advocacy group.

At the same time, the FDA's supplement division is understaffed and underfunded, with about 60 people and a budget of only $10 million to police a $19.4 billion-a-year industry. To regulate drugs, annual sales of which are 12 times the amount of supplement sales, the FDA has

The standards for demonstrating a supplement is hazardous are so high that it can take the FDA years to build a case.

almost 43 times as much money and almost 48 times as many people.

"The law has never been fully funded," said William Hubbard, FDA associate commissioner for policy and planning. "There's never been the resources to do all the things the law would command us to do."

The agency has learned that it must tread carefully

Twelve supplements you should avoid

The 12 supplement ingredients in this table have been linked to serious adverse events or, in the case of glandular supplements, to strong theoretical risks. They're all readily available on the Web, where our shoppers bought them both individually and in multi-ingredient "combination products."

We think it's wise to avoid all of them. But the strength of that warning varies with the strength of the evidence and the size of the risk. So we've divided the dirty dozen into three categories: definitely hazardous, very likely hazardous, and likely hazardous.

Name (Also known as)	Dangers	Regulatory actions
DEFINITELY HAZARDOUS Documented organ failure and known carcinogenic properties		
Aristolochic acid (Aristolochia, birthwort, snakeroot, snakeweed, sangree root, sangrel, serpentary, serpentaria; asarum canadense, wild ginger). Can be an ingredient in Chinese herbal products labeled fang ji, mu tong, ma dou ling, and mu xiang. Can be an unlabeled substitute for other herbs, including akebia, asarum, clematis, cocculus, stephania, and vladimiria species.	Potent human carcinogen; kidney failure, sometimes requiring transplant; deaths reported.	FDA warning to consumers and industry and import alert in April 2001. Banned in 7 European countries and Egypt, Japan, and Venezuela.
VERY LIKELY HAZARDOUS Banned in other countries, FDA warning, or adverse effects in studies		
Androstenedione (4-androstene-3, 17-dione, andro, androstene)	Increased cancer risk, decrease in HDL cholesterol.	FDA warned 23 companies to stop manufacturing, marketing, and distributing in March 2004. Banned by athletic associations.
Comfrey (Symphytum officinale, ass ear, black root, blackwort, bruisewort, consolidae radix, consound, gum plant, healing herb, knitback, knitbone, salsify, slippery root, symphytum radix, wallwort)	Abnormal liver function or damage, often irreversible; deaths reported.	FDA advised industry to remove from market in July 2001.
Chaparral (Larrea divaricata, creosote bush, greasewood, hediondilla, jarilla, larreastat)	Abnormal liver function or damage, often irreversible; deaths reported.	FDA warning to consumers in December 1992.
Germander (Teucrium chamaedrys, wall germander, wild germander)	Abnormal liver function or damage, often irreversible; deaths reported.	Banned in France and Germany.
Kava (Piper methysticum, ava, awa, gea, gi, intoxicating pepper, kao, kavain, kawa-pfeffer, kew, long pepper, malohu, maluk, meruk, milik, rauschpfeffer, sakau, tonga, wurzelstock, yagona, yangona)	Abnormal liver function or damage, occasionally irreversible; deaths reported.	FDA warning to consumers in March 2002. Banned in Canada, Germany, Singapore, South Africa, and Switzerland.

when regulating supplements. The first time it tried to regulate the dangerous stimulant ephedra, in 1997, overwhelming opposition from Congress and industry forced it to back down.

As a result, the FDA is sometimes left practicing what Silverglade calls "regulation by press release"—issuing warnings about dangerous supplements and hoping that consumers and health practitioners read them.

There are signs of hope. The FDA has said that if the ban on ephedra holds up against likely legal challenges, it plans to go after other harmful supplements. Federal legislation has recently been introduced to strengthen the FDA's authority under DSHEA and give the agency more money to enforce the act.

But the supplement marketplace still holds hidden hazards for consumers, especially among products that aren't in the headlines. "Consumers are provided with more information about the composition and nutritional value of a loaf of bread than about the ingredients and potential hazards of botanical medicines," said Arthur Grollman, M.D., professor of pharmacological sciences at the State University of New York, Stony Brook, and a critic of DSHEA.

A QUESTION OF SAFETY

Supplement-industry advocates say the ephedra ban

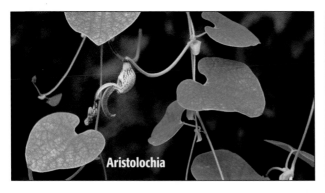

Aristolochia

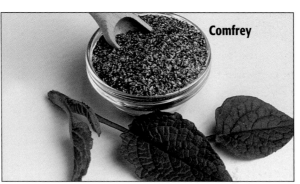

Comfrey

Name (Also known as)	Dangers	Regulatory actions
LIKELY HAZARDOUS Adverse-event reports or theoretical risks		
Bitter orange (Citrus aurantium, green orange, kijitsu, neroli oil, Seville orange, shangzhou zhiqiao, sour orange, zhi oiao, zhi xhi)	High blood pressure; increased risk of heart arrythmias, heart attack, stroke.	None
Lobelia (Lobelia inflata, asthma weed, bladderpod, emetic herb, gagroot, lobelie, indian tobacco, pukeweed, vomit wort, wild tobacco)	Breathing difficulty, rapid heartbeat, low blood pressure, diarrhea, dizziness, tremors; possible deaths reported.	Banned in Bangladesh and Italy.
Organ/glandular extracts (brain/adrenal/pituitary/placenta/other gland "substance" or "concentrate")	Theoretical risk of mad cow disease, particularly from brain extracts.	FDA banned high-risk bovine materials from older cows in food supplements in January 2004. (High-risk parts from cows under 30 months still permitted.) Banned in France and Switzerland.
Pennyroyal oil (Hedeoma pulegioides, lurk-in-the-ditch, mosquito plant, piliolerial, pudding grass, pulegium, run-by-the-ground, squaw balm, squawmint, stinking balm, tickweed)	Liver and kidney failure, nerve damage, convulsions, abdominal tenderness, burning of the throat; deaths reported.	None
Scullcap (Scutellaria lateriflora, blue pimpernel, helmet flower, hoodwort, mad weed, mad-dog herb, mad-dog weed, quaker bonnet, scutelluria, skullcap)	Abnormal liver function or damage.	None
Yohimbe (Pausinystalia yohimbe, johimbi, yohimbehe, yohimbine)	Change in blood pressure, heart arrythmias, respiratory depression, heart attack; deaths reported.	None

Sources: Natural Medicines Comprehensive Database 2004 and Consumers Union's medical and research consultants. (Originally appeared in the May 2004 issue of CONSUMER REPORTS.)

What you can do

While legislation regarding the supplement industry is pending in Congress, you cannot rely on the federal government to ensure that dietary supplements are safe and effective. Here are some steps you can take to minimize your risk from any supplements you decide to take:

• Stay away from the dirty dozen. All carry risks that in our view are unacceptable. In combination products, you need to read the detailed ingredient list in the tiny print on the back. Who could otherwise guess, for instance, that Gaia Herbs' PMS Day 14-28 capsules contain kava? (To the company's credit, the label includes a warning about liver toxicity.)

• Do not take daily doses of vitamins and minerals that exceed the safe upper limits. While vitamins and minerals are by far the safest and best-studied of supplements, it's possible to overdose on some of them. Recommended allowances and safe upper limits can be found online at *www.ific.org/publications/other/driupdateom.cfm.*

• Limit your intake of other supplements. Over the years, our medical and nutritional consultants have identified and tested a few products, other than standard multivitamins, with possible benefits and sufficiently low risks to recommend for general use: saw palmetto for benign enlarged prostate in men, glucosamine and chondroitin for arthritis, and fish-oil capsules (omega-3 fatty acids) for heart disease. (We plan to test additional supplements with potential benefits, such as probiotics.)

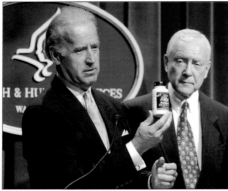

U.S. Senators Joseph Biden (left) and Orrin Hatch were on hand when the FDA announced its ban on ephedra in December 2003.

• Tell your doctor about your supplements. "The Achilles' heel of unregulated supplements is the risk created by herb-prescription drug interactions," said Grollman, the pharmacologist at the State University of New York. "St. John's wort, used to treat depression, for instance, may reduce the effectiveness of prescription drugs used by millions of Americans for hypertension, AIDS, heart failure, asthma, and other chronic diseases."

• Stay away from supplements for weight control. These products frequently contain several stimulants that have never been adequately tested separately, let alone in combinations. "I'd just as soon experiment with rats first rather than using the U.S. population as guinea pigs," said Bill Gurley, Ph.D., professor of pharmaceutical sciences at the University of Arkansas.

• Do your own research. Health-food-store clerks and marketers, alternative-medicine practitioners, herbal company Web sites, and even physicians are not necessarily knowledgeable about the scientific evidence regarding dietary supplements. These two Web sites contain reliable information: the National Institutes of Health site at *ods.od.nih.gov/databases/ibids.html* and Memorial Sloan-Kettering Cancer Center's site at *www.mskcc.org/mskcc/html/11570.cfm.*

• Watch for adverse events. Let your doctor know if you experience anything worrisome after starting a supplement. If your doctor concludes that the side effect may be related to the supplement, be sure to report it to the FDA, by calling 800-332-1088 or by visiting *www.fda.gov/medwatch.*

---

demonstrates that DSHEA gives the FDA enough power to protect consumers from unsafe products. "I don't think there's anything wrong except that FDA has only recently begun vigorous and active enforcement of the law," said Annette Dickinson, Ph.D., president of the Council for Responsible Nutrition, a major trade association for the supplement industry.

However, critics of DSHEA think the ban illustrates the extremes to which the FDA must go to outlaw a hazardous product.

When the agency initially tried to rein in ephedra use in 1997, after receiving hundreds of reports of adverse events, it sought not an outright ban but dosage restrictions and sterner warning labels. The industry mounted a furious counter-attack, including the creation of a public-relations group called the Ephedra Education Council and a scientific review from a private consulting firm, commissioned by Dickinson's trade group, that concluded ephedra was safe. After the U.S. General Accounting Office said the FDA "did not establish a causal link" between taking ephedra and deaths or injuries, the agency was forced to drop its proposal.

The industry continued to vigorously market and defend ephedra. Metabolife International, a leading ephedra manufacturer, did not let the FDA know that it had received 14,684 complaints of adverse events associ-

Drug labels must mention possible adverse effects, but supplement makers don't have to disclose safety warnings.

ated with its ephedra product, Metabolife 356, in the previous five years, including 18 heart attacks, 26 strokes, 43 seizures, and 5 deaths. It took the pressure of congressional and Justice Department investigations to get the company to turn over the complaints in 2002. Then Steve Bechler, a pitcher for the Baltimore Orioles, died unexpectedly in 2003 while taking another ephedra supplement, Xenadrine RFA-1. With sales suffering from the bad publicity, manufacturers began to replace ephedra with other stimulants such as bitter orange, which mimics ephedra in chemical composition and function.

"All of a sudden Congress dropped objections to an ephedra ban and started demanding the FDA act," said Silverglade.

To amass the necessary scientific evidence that it hoped would satisfy the demanding standard set by DSHEA, the FDA took aggressive action: It commissioned an outside review from the RAND Corporation, analyzed adverse-event reports, and pored over every available shred of scientific evidence.

"We've gone the whole nine yards to collect and evaluate all the possible evidence," Mark McClellan, commissioner of the FDA, said in announcing the ban. "We will be doing our best to defend this in court, and if that's not sufficient, it may be time to re-examine the act."

DRUGS VS. SUPPLEMENTS

In an October 2002 nationwide Harris Poll of 1,010 adults, 59 percent of respondents said they believed that supplements must be approved by a government agency before they can be sold to the public. Sixty-eight percent said the government requires warning labels on supplements' potential side effects or dangers. Fifty-five percent said supplement manufacturers can't make safety claims without solid scientific support.

They were wrong. None of those protections exist for supplements—only for prescription and over-the-counter medicines. Here are the major differences in the safety regulations:

Testing for hazards. Before approval, drugs must be proved effective, with an acceptable safety profile, by means of lab research and rigorous human clinical trials involving a minimum of several thousand people, many millions of dollars, and several years.

In contrast, supplement manufacturers can introduce new products without any testing for safety and efficacy. The maker's only obligation is to send the FDA a copy of the language on the label.

"Products regulated by DSHEA were presumed to be safe because of their long history of use, often in other countries," said Jane E. Henney, M.D., commissioner of the FDA from 1998 to 2001. "As their use dramatically increased in this country after the passage of DSHEA, the presumption of safety may have been misplaced, particularly for products other than traditional vitamins and minerals. Some, like ephedra, act like drugs and thus have similar risks."

The only exceptions to this "presumption of safety" are supplement ingredients that weren't being sold in the U.S. when DSHEA took effect. Makers of such "new dietary ingredients" must show the FDA evidence of the products' safety before marketing them. The FDA invoked that rarely used provision in its action against androstenedione. After years of allowing andro to be marketed without restriction, the agency declared that it was "not aware" that the supplement was used before DSHEA, so it couldn't be sold without evidence of safety.

Disclosing the risks. Drug labels and package inserts

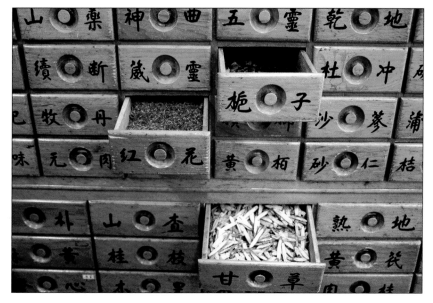

Reporting the problems. By law, drug companies are required to tell the FDA about any reports of product-related adverse events that they receive from any source. Almost every year, drugs are removed from the market based on safety risks that first surfaced in those reports.

In contrast, supplement makers don't have to report adverse events. Indeed, in the five years after DSHEA took effect, 1994 to 1999, fewer than 10 of the more than 2,500 reports that the FDA received came from manufacturers, according to a 2001 estimate from the inspector general of the U.S. Department of Health and Human Services. (Other sources of reports included consumers, health practitioners, and poison-control centers.) Overall, the FDA estimates that it learns of less than 1 percent of adverse events involving dietary supplements.

must mention all possible adverse effects and interactions. But supplement makers don't have to put safety warnings on the labels, even for products with known serious hazards.

We bought a product called Relaxit whose label had no warning about the kava it contained, even though the American Herbal Products Association, an industry trade group, recommends a detailed, though voluntary warning label about potential liver toxicity on all kava products.

Natural does not equal safe. Poisonous mushrooms are natural.

Ensuring product quality. Drugs must conform to "good manufacturing practices" that guarantee that their contents are pure and in the quantities stated on the label. While DSHEA gave the FDA authority to impose similar standards on supplements, it took until 2003 for the agency to propose regulations—as yet not final—to implement that part of the law.

Contaminants, too, regularly turn up in supplements. In 1998 Richard Ko, Ph.D., of the California Department of Health Services reported that 32 percent of the Asian patent medicines he tested contained pharmaceuticals or heavy metals that weren't on the label. In 2002, the FDA oversaw a voluntary manufacturer recall of a "prostate health" supplement called PC SPES that, according to tests by the California department, contained a powerful prescription blood thinner, warfarin.

THE "NATURAL" MYSTIQUE

Many makers market their supplements as "natural," exploiting assumptions that such products can't harm you. That's a dangerous assumption, said Lois Swirsky Gold, Ph.D., director of the Carcinogenic Potency Project at the University of California, Berkeley, and an expert on chemical carcinogens. "Natural is hemlock, natural is arsenic, natural is poisonous mushrooms," she said.

A cautionary example is aristolochic acid, which occurs naturally in species of Aristolochia vines that grow wild in many parts of the world. In addition to being a powerful kidney toxin, it is on the World Health Organization's list of human carcinogens. "It's one of the most potent chemicals of 1,400 in my Carcinogenic Potency Database," Gold said. "People have taken high doses similar to the doses that animals are given in tests, and they both get tumors very quickly."

The dangers of aristolochic acid have been known since at least 1993, when medical-journal articles began appearing about 105 patrons of a Belgian weight-loss clinic who had suffered kidney failure after consuming Chinese herbs adulterated with Aristolochia. At least 18 of the women also subsequently developed cancer near the kidney.

These findings prompted the FDA to issue a nationwide warning against Aristolochia in 2001 and to impose a ban on further imports of the herb. But in early 2004, more than two years after the import ban went into effect, CONSUMER REPORTS was able to purchase products online that were labeled as containing Aristolochia. In 2003, Gold identified more than 100 products for sale online with botanical ingredients listed by the FDA as known or suspected to contain aristolochic acid.

Donna Andrade-Wheaton, a former aerobics instructor in Rhode Island, learned those facts too late to save her kidneys. After taking Chinese herbs containing Aristolochia for more than two years, she suffered severe kidney damage; her kidney tissues were found to contain aristolochic acid. In late 2002, at age 39, she underwent a kidney transplant.

Andrade-Wheaton is suing both the acupuncturist who gave her the herbs and several companies that manufactured them. The acupuncturist declined to discuss the case on the record, and the manufacturer did not return our phone calls.

There's another widespread and false assumption about natural supplements: that they're always pure, unprocessed products of the earth. Because DSHEA permits the marketing of concentrates and extracts, supplement makers can and do manipulate ingredients to increase the concentrations of pharmacologically active compounds.

That's especially true of the many weight-loss supplements designed for "thermogenic" stimulant effects—boosting calorie expenditure by revving the metabolic rate.

On one Internet shopping tour, for instance, we bought a product called Thermorexin—"the Hottest new Thermogenic on the market!" Its label

Keep in mind that there's virtually no regulation of the herbal products sold by bulk or in pills.

says it contains, among its 22 ingredients, 30 milligrams of theophylline derived from a black tea extract and the stimulant bitter orange. Sold as Theo-Dur and other brands, theophylline is a prescription drug and an effective asthma treatment, but most doctors seldom prescribe it because it can cause seizures and irregular heartbeats at relatively low doses.

Larry Berube, president of Anafit, Thermorexin's manufacturer, based in Orlando, Fla., described how the product's combination of ingredients was developed: "Once we find out that the FDA says it's OK, we put them together in the lab, run our tests, and do our trials, and if it comes up good, we capsulate it, put it online and in the stores and sell it," he said.

Those tests involved asking fitness professionals to use the supplement, and measuring their heart rate and blood pressure, Berube said. The company doesn't use a control group, he said. Then "we go to the fitness discussion boards and let trainers and people know we have a new product and do they want to try it," he said. "And then they try it, and they report back." Berube said he has not heard of any bad reactions to Thermorexin.

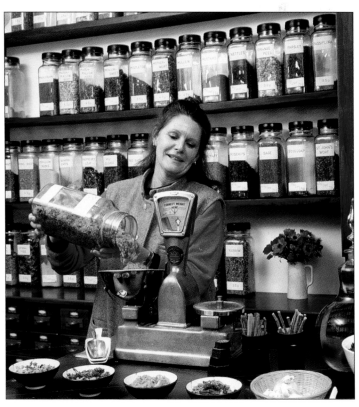

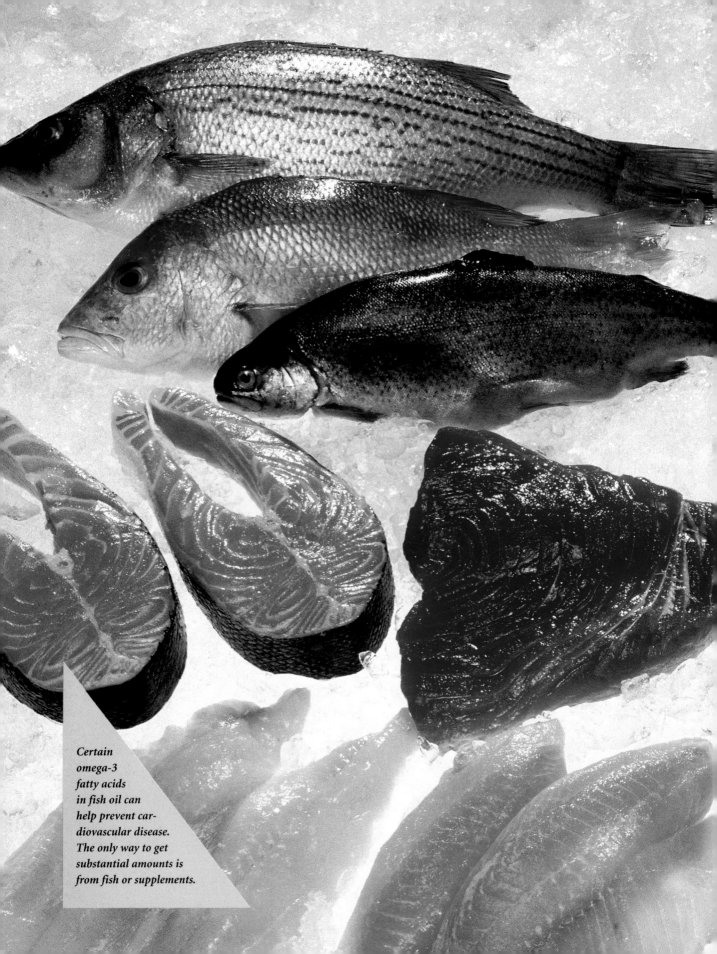

Certain omega-3 fatty acids in fish oil can help prevent cardiovascular disease. The only way to get substantial amounts is from fish or supplements.

Omega-3 oil: fish or pills?

A flood of scientific findings on fish oil points to a startling conclusion: Certain omega-3 fatty acids in the oil, consumed either from fish or fish-oil capsules, appear to offer as much protection against dying from coronary heart disease as do cholesterol-lowering drugs.

The evidence of fish oil's protective powers is so strong that the American Heart Association now urges everyone to eat at least two small 3-ounce servings of fish a week. That's particularly important after menopause in women and after age 45 or so in men, when coronary risk starts to rise.

In 2002 the heart association advised people who already have heart disease to consume about 1 gram a day of the active ingredients in fish oil—omega-3s called EPA and DHA. To follow that recommendation, the average person would have to take at least some fish-oil pills. This is one of the few times that a major health organization has endorsed any dietary supplement for treating or preventing disease.

But consumers who want the coronary protection that those omega-3s can provide may have other questions:

• **Who else needs the pills?** Millions of Americans have increased coronary risk but no apparent heart disease. Our medical consultants say that fish-oil supplements may make sense for those people as well, depending on the extent of their risk for heart disease.

• **Is fish safe?** Young children and women who are nursing or pregnant or who may become pregnant should avoid or limit their intake of certain types of fish that can be contaminated, notably with mercury. Other people should vary their choices, frequently eat the species unlikely to contain contaminants (see "Right fish, least risk," on page 46), and sharply restrict their intake of the species with the most mercury, namely shark, swordfish, and king mackerel.

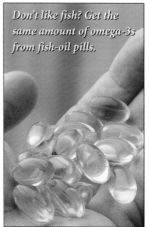

Don't like fish? Get the same amount of omega-3s from fish-oil pills.

• **Are fish-oil supplements safe and are their contents reliable?** The federal Food and Drug Administration rarely monitors the composition and purity of dietary supplements. But our tests of 16 top-selling fish-oil supplements were reassuring: All those pills contained roughly as much EPA and DHA as their labels promised. None showed evidence of spoilage, and none contained significant amounts of mercury, the worrisome PCBs, or dioxin.

So the choice boils down to price, and we found good news there, too: Two brands, Kirkland Signature Natural Fish Oil and Member's Mark Omega 3 Fish Oil, each a CR Best Buy, supplied the desirable daily dosage for less than half to as little as a tenth of the cost of the other brands we tested.

FIVE-WAY PROTECTION

Studies suggest several possible mechanisms to explain how fish oil helps minimize the consequences of heart disease and perhaps prevent the disease in the first place:

• It may electrically stabilize the heart-muscle cells,

reducing the likelihood that a heart attack will trigger an arrhythmia or potentially deadly heartbeat disturbance.

- It may fight inflammation, which makes arterial plaque deposits more likely to break apart, create blood clots, and thus trigger a heart attack.
- It may make certain blood cells less sticky and less likely to form clots.
- It may make the arteries more elastic, reducing the chance that increased blood pressure will cause plaque deposits to rupture.
- High doses can reduce blood levels of triglycerides, a fat that may increase heart-disease risk.

A DRAMATIC DROP IN DEATHS

The benefits of fish oil emerged when researchers noticed that people who ate fish frequently suffered fewer heart attacks and died of heart disease at a lower rate than those who seldom ate fish. Most significant, those studies showed that eating fish offers powerful protection against one of the most dreaded and unpredictable consequences of heart disease: "sudden-death" heart attacks that kill within minutes. Subsequent research suggested that high fish consumption may also reduce the risk of stroke.

Controlled clinical trials have confirmed that a steady diet of fish or fish-oil supplements works as "secondary prevention," reducing the likelihood of a repeat heart attack in people who've already had a first attack.

For example, the Diet and Reinfarction Trial, involving some 2,000 heart-attack survivors in Wales, found that those who increased their EPA and DHA intake from fish by at least 500 milligrams a day for two years had a 29 percent lower death rate than those who didn't boost their fish intake; a drop in fatal heart attacks accounted for that entire benefit. But another trial, involving some 11,300 Italian heart-attack survivors followed for 3½ years, found that those given 850 mil-

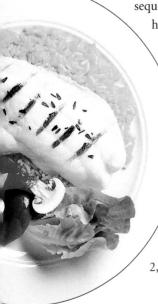

People with normal heart risk should eat fish twice a week.

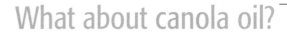

What about canola oil?

Fish is the only food that directly supplies substantial amounts of the omega-3 fatty acids EPA and DHA. But you can get them indirectly from vegetable oils rich in another omega-3, alpha-linolenic acid, which the body converts to EPA and DHA. Flaxseed oil contains the most alpha-linolenic acid; canola, olive, soybean, and walnut oil contain moderate amounts. Researchers aren't certain how much alpha-linolenic gets converted, but it's almost surely less than 15 percent, probably much less.

Nevertheless, several population studies suggest that people whose diet supplies a lot of alpha-linolenic acid may suffer fewer fatal heart attacks than others. So far, researchers have not clearly determined whether alpha-linolenic supplementation can reduce coronary risk.

Based on the available evidence, the American Heart Association advises everyone not only to consume fish or fish oil regularly, depending on their coronary risk, but also to prepare meals using oils rich in alpha-linolenic acid.

ligrams a day of EPA and DHA from supplements had 20 percent fewer deaths overall and 45 percent fewer sudden-death heart attacks than the untreated control group.

Long-term clinical trials of fish-oil supplements have not yet been conducted in people who have major risk factors for heart disease, such as diabetes or high blood pressure, but who haven't developed any apparent signs of the disease. So researchers cannot be sure that taking these supplements would work as "primary prevention"—keeping a heart attack from occurring in the first place.

William S. Harris, Ph.D., of the University of Missouri and director of the Lipid and Metabolic Research Laboratory at the MidAmerica Heart Institute, notes, "There has never been a cardiologic treatment that worked as secondary prevention that didn't also work as primary prevention."

CR quick recommendations

We found no significant differences in the quality or purity of these supplements. So choose them based on price. The two least-expensive products we tested are sold only at warehouse clubs: Kirkland Signature Natural Fish Oil (1) at Costco and Member's Mark Omega 3 Fish Oil (2) at Sam's Club. For a daily dose of about 1 gram of EPA and DHA combined—the amounts recommended for people with heart disease—those products cost at least $44 a year less than their nearest competitor in price. That savings will roughly pay for the annual membership fee of $45 at Costco, $35 at Sam's Club.

If you don't have one of those clubs near you or don't want to join, you can order Kirkland Signature over the Internet at generally higher prices but without the annual fee. For example, we found a year's supply for about $43, including shipping, at *www.mypatienteducation.com*; that's still less expensive than any products we tested that are sold outside the clubs. You can order a minimum of a year's

worth, since the capsules should remain unspoiled for at least that long after they were manufactured, provided you keep them out of direct sunlight. But check the expiration date to be sure. Refrigerating or freezing the supplements should prolong their shelf life.

For optimal use of fish-oil pills, follow these guidelines:

● To get roughly the clinical-trial dosage of EPA and DHA, take the number of pills listed in our table. In several cases that number differs from the number or range on the label. That's because the manufacturer recommended a higher or lower dosage than was used in the most compelling clinical trials.

● The pills may cause some initial side effects, such as bloating and burping up a "fishy" taste. Freezing the capsules before taking them may minimize those effects.

● For heart benefits, it doesn't seem to matter whether you take the daily capsules all at once or separately. But taking them with meals might decrease any side effects.

Fish-oil pills Ratings
In price order.

	Product, in price order	Pills per day	Cost per day	Cost per year
1	**Kirkland Signature** Natural Fish Oil (Costco) **CR Best Buy**	3	$0.06	$22
2	**Member's Mark** Omega 3 Fish Oil (Sam's Club) **CR Best Buy**	3	0.06	22
3	**Spring Valley** Natural Fish Oil Concentrate	3	0.18	66
4	**Walgreens** Fish Oil Concentrate	4	0.24	88
5	**Vitasmart** Naturals Fish Oil Concentrate (Kmart)	4	0.28	100
6	**CVS Pharmacy** Natural Fish Oil Concentrate	3	0.30	110
7	**Natrol** Omega-3	4	0.32	117
8	**Sundown** Fish Oil	4	0.32	117
9	**GNC** Fish Body Oils	4	0.36	131
10	**Nature's Bounty** Salmon Oil	5	0.40	146
11	**Rite Aid** Natural Fish Oil	4	0.40	146
12	**YourLife** Natural Fish Oil Concentrate	3	0.42	153
13	**Country Life** Natural Omega-3 Fish Body Oils	4	0.48	175
14	**Eckerd** Natural Fish Oil Concentrate	4	0.52	190
15	**Spectrum Essentials** Omega 3 Norwegian Fish Oil	4	0.52	190
16	**Solgar** Omega-3 "700"	2	0.60	219

This chart originally appeared in the July 2003 issue of CONSUMER REPORTS.

GUIDE TO THE RATINGS We tested all 16 products in our laboratories for the omega-3s EPA and DHA. And we commissioned two independent labs to test them for mercury, dioxin, dioxin-like PCBs, and decomposition. **Pills per day** is the number of pills needed to obtain close to 1 gram of EPA and DHA combined, the daily dose recommended by the American Heart Association for people with heart disease. **Cost per day**, based on the approximate retail prices of the largest available bottles, gives the daily cost of the number of pills needed to supply close to the American Heart Association's recommended daily dose. **Cost per year** gives the cost of taking those daily doses for 1 year.

Right fish, least risk

Fish is rich in omega-3s and other nutrients. But some species may contain excessive amounts of certain pollutants. The most comprehensive data on those pollutants involve mercury. Last spring, two federal agencies issued the government's first advisory on limits for safe amounts of tuna to eat, because of its mercury content. The Food and Drug Administration and the Environmental Protection Agency say that women of childbearing age, pregnant women, nursing mothers, and young children should eat no more than 6 ounces of tuna steak or canned white albacore tuna per week. (Albacore, different from light tuna, is more likely to accumulate mercury.) As a result of industrial pollution and power-plant emissions, mercury accumulates in fish as they feed and can harm developing nervous systems.

But the government's advice is at odds with a longstanding EPA safety assessment, which suggests that the limit should be just 3 ounces of albacore a week. That's the amount recommended by the food-safety experts at Consumers Union, publisher of CONSUMER REPORTS. They say that if women of childbearing age eat albacore, any other fish they eat that week should be very low-mercury (see the table, right). We recommend that young children not eat albacore at all.

Ads from the U.S. Tuna Foundation, a trade group, try to put the government advisory in a very rosy light. One ad says, among other things, that mercury levels in albacore are "well below government standards." But the government has set no safety standards for mercury in albacore or any other fish.

The government's advisory said that women of childbearing age and young children should not eat king mackerel, shark, swordfish, or tilefish. However, they may eat up to 12 ounces a week of lower-mercury fish. Fish sticks and fish sandwiches typically served in restaurants are made from low-mercury fish.

Seafood	Mercury (parts per million)
Light Tuna	0.12
Albacore	0.35
Clams	
Oysters	
Pickerel	undetectable
Shrimp	
Whiting	
Fresh or frozen salmon	
Tilapia	0.01
Sardines	0.02
Freshwater trout	0.03
Anchovies	0.04
Catfish	
Flounder	
Mullet	0.05
Scallops	
Sole	
Blue, King, Snow crab	
Pollock	0.06
American shad	
Squid	0.07
Whitefish	

Women of childbearing age should choose from the very low-mercury alternatives to tuna listed here. Young children who eat four or more 3-ounce servings of fish a week should be served only types with a mercury concentration of less than 0.05 parts per million. Light tuna contains 0.12 ppm of mercury; albacore, 0.35 ppm. Chart originally appeared in the July 2004 issue of CONSUMER REPORTS.

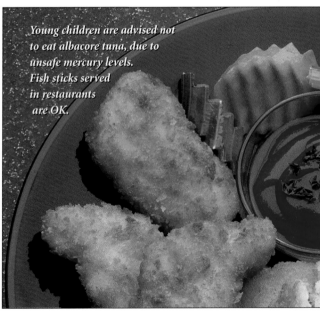

Young children are advised not to eat albacore tuna, due to unsafe mercury levels. Fish sticks served in restaurants are OK.

Revived hope for fighting fat: CLA

The latest research has bolstered the case for conjugated linoleic acid (CLA), the polyunsaturated "wonder fat" that supposedly makes you leaner.

Although animal studies suggest that CLA supplements may reduce body fat, increase muscle mass, or both, research in humans until now has been considerably less encouraging. But results from the largest and longest trial to date, published in June 2004, suggest that CLA may yet fulfill its fat-fighting promise.

Norwegian researchers randomly assigned 180 healthy overweight volunteers to take 4.5-gram supplements of CLA or placebo pills; they received general advice about diet and exercise, but no specific regimens. After a year body fat and muscle stayed constant in the placebo group, but the CLA group lost an average of 7 percent of total body fat and boosted muscle mass by 1.5 percent.

Overall the CLA group lost an average of only 3 pounds. But replacing fat with muscle might make you look slimmer even if you didn't lose weight. And the slight increase in muscle mass could be important because most weight-loss agents reduce muscle as well as fat.

Some researchers theorize that CLA may work by drawing fat out of the body's fat cells or by inhibiting their incorporation of further fat, thereby redirecting calories into muscle cells.

Despite those promising findings, further study is needed before CLA can be recommended as a fat-fighting pill. The shift in the muscle-to-fat ratio was modest and of uncertain clinical and cosmetic significance. Moreover, the CLA group experienced an increase in lipoprotein(a), a cholesterol-like substance linked to increased heart risk. And the safety and efficacy of CLA has not been studied in people with obesity-related conditions, such as diabetes, heart disease, and hypertension.

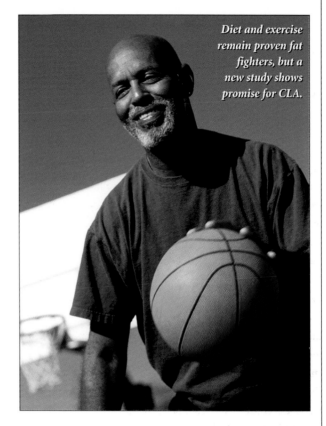

Diet and exercise remain proven fat fighters, but a new study shows promise for CLA.

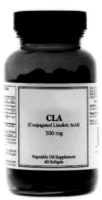

CLA
(Conjugated Linoleic Acid)
500 mg

Vegetable Oil Supplement
60 Softgels

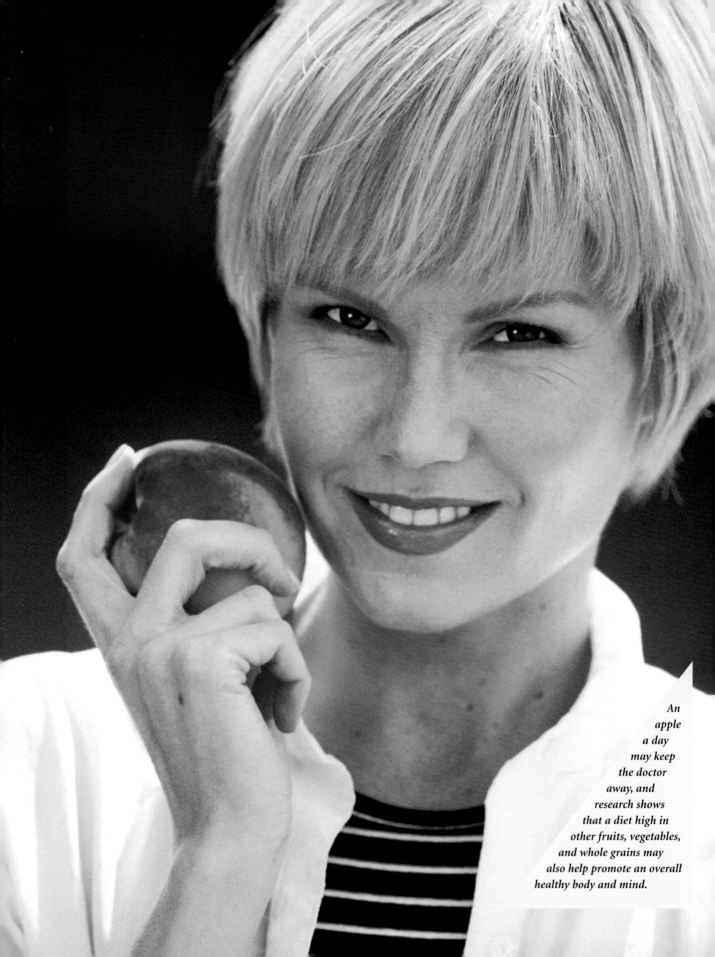

An apple a day may keep the doctor away, and research shows that a diet high in other fruits, vegetables, and whole grains may also help promote an overall healthy body and mind.

Food for thought:

Can meals and supplements make you smarter and happier?

We all know intuitively that what we eat can influence how we think and feel. "Just consider an inconsolable, irritable baby who, immediately after nursing, turns calm and responsive," notes Simon Young, Ph.D., a behavioral neurochemist at McGill University in Montreal. But exactly which kinds of meals, foods, and supplements can sharpen your thinking or lift your spirits—or dull and dampen them?

The 10-question quiz below will test your knowledge of the links between diet, thought, and mood. The answers on the following pages will untangle what's really known from what's merely conjecture—or just plain wrong.

QUESTIONS

1. Dietary supplements, such as ginkgo, can help compensate for normal age-related declines in memory. **True or False?**

2. Dietary supplements, such as St. John's wort and SAM-e, can improve your mood. **True or False?**

3. The dietary steps that help protect your heart can also help keep your brain sharp as you age. **True or False?**

4. Low intake of B vitamins can cause mental decline. **True or False?**

5. Eating lots of sugar makes kids inattentive and overactive. **True or False?**

6. Cake, pasta, and other high-carbohydrate foods can help some people feel calm. **True or False?**

7. High-carb foods can help you think more clearly. **True or False?**

8. Eating breakfast boosts cognitive performance. **True or False?**

9. Eating lunch boosts cognitive performance. **True or False?**

10. Consuming lots of caffeine is a good way to sharpen your thinking. **True or False?**

ANSWERS

1. Supplements can boost memory.

False. Supplements aren't likely to improve cognitive performance in most people. The most popular "brain-enhancing" supplement is the herb ginkgo biloba, which is commonly used in Europe to treat dementia. In this country, the National Institute on Aging is funding a clinical trial of ginkgo as a treatment for Alzheimer's disease. Other supplements touted for their cognitive potential include acetyl-L-carnitine, phosphatidylserine, and vinpocetine. Many products combine two or more of those substances.

But two recent scientific reviews—one on ginkgo, one on the other supplements—concluded that the studies so far were so small or poorly designed that it's impossible to know what effect, if any, the supplements have in treating dementia or preventing memory loss. Even in individual studies of ginkgo that did show a benefit, the review said the improvements were slight—even less than what you'd expect from a glucose drink (see answer 7 on page 52) or listening to a stimulating story.

"We know that simply exercising your mind—reading good books, learning new games or languages—is an excellent way to preserve mental acuity," says Paul Gold, Ph.D., a psychology professor at the University of Illinois at Urbana-Champaign and author of the recent ginkgo review. "It's not as easy as popping a pill, but you'll get more out of it."

2. Supplements can improve mood.

True. But dietary supplements are likely to help only mild or moderate emotional problems.

Several clinical trials have shown that two popular supplements—extracts of the herb St. John's wort and

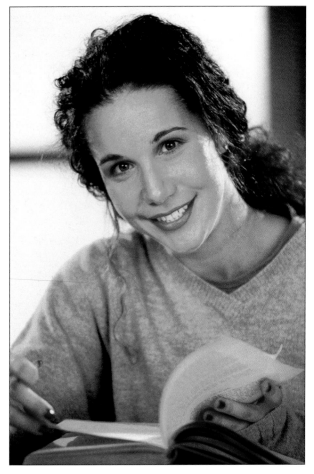

Reading is one type of mental exercise to help you stay sharp.

s-adenosyl-methionine (SAM-e), a substance that boosts serotonin levels—relieve mild depression as effectively as a prescription antidepressant.

However, there's no evidence that those products help tame severe emotional problems; in fact, one recent clinical trial found that St. John's wort does not relieve major depression. Whether these products have any effect on garden-variety sadness or nervousness is not known, mainly because standard tests aren't sensitive enough to detect any possible impact on temporary bad moods. These remedies almost certainly will not improve a normal, undisturbed mood.

While prescription antidepressant and antianxiety drugs often cause side effects, these "natural" supplements can pose risks, too.

St. John's wort can cause sun sensitivity and decrease the effectiveness of a host of other medications, including

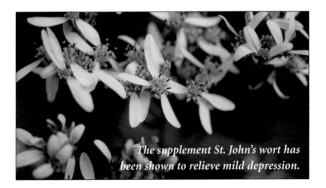

The supplement St. John's wort has been shown to relieve mild depression.

oral contraceptives, cholesterol-lowering "statin" drugs, and certain blood-pressure drugs. SAM-e can cause nervousness, insomnia, and possibly mania. Neither product should be taken with another antidepressant, since the herb and possibly SAM-e can magnify the medication's effects and side effects.

If you're considering using either substance, first talk to a mental-health professional, who can distinguish a mild or moderate problem from a more serious one, which requires prescription medication, psychotherapy, or both. Milder problems could possibly be treated with either St. John's wort or SAM-e, though a health professional should check for drug interactions and monitor your progress.

3. Diets that help the heart help the brain.

True. The brain consumes roughly 20 percent of the oxygen you breathe. So anything that threatens the ability of the heart or blood vessels to circulate oxygen-rich blood also threatens the brain's health and function. Indeed, studies suggest that much of the decline in cognitive power results from a decreased supply of oxygen to the brain.

A diet low in saturated fat and cholesterol can help keep plaque deposits from forming in the arteries. Eating plenty of fruits, vegetables, grains, and low-fat dairy products not only tends to minimize your intake of fat and cholesterol but also supplies numerous nutrients that help keep the arteries healthy. Exercising and stopping smoking will also protect the brain, by improving cardiovascular function.

4. Lack of B vitamins can dull the mind.

True. Researchers have long known that a gross deficiency of vitamin B12 can cause a certain type of dementia, and that correcting the deficiency can sometimes restore clear thinking. However, recent research suggests that even moderate deficiencies of B12 or folic acid (another B

vitamin) may contribute to cognitive decline and possibly the onset of Alzheimer's disease, probably by elevating levels of the amino acid homocysteine. Other evidence links low levels of B vitamins or high homocysteine levels with an increased risk of depression. To help explain those findings, laboratory studies show that homocysteine inhibits the growth of new brain cells and may interfere with the metabolism of certain brain chemicals that help regulate mood and memory. In addition, folic acid and vitamins B6 and B12 help preserve the brain by preserving the cerebral arteries.

While a diet high in grains, produce, and low-fat dairy products generally provides plenty of the three Bs, many older people don't secrete enough stomach acid to extract and absorb vitamin B12 from unfortified food. So everyone over age 50 should take a modest daily B12 supplement or consume B12-fortified foods, notably breakfast cereals.

Note that folic acid may further protect against mental decline by maintaining adequate supplies of choline, a nutrient that helps control homocysteine and is a precursor to acetylcholine and other brain chemicals. While most people obtain enough choline from their diet, the body uses folic acid to create choline when the level dips too low. Choline's essential role in brain function is one reason why the Food and Drug Administration has started allowing manufacturers to label certain foods as high in choline.

5. Sugar makes kids hyperactive.

False. The number of children with attention deficit hyperactivity disorder does seem to have soared in recent years. And the simultaneous rise in kids' sugar consumption seems to support the common, persistent belief that sugar makes kids "bounce off the walls." But the apparent epidemic of overactivity almost surely stems solely from increased diagnosis, caused by heightened awareness of

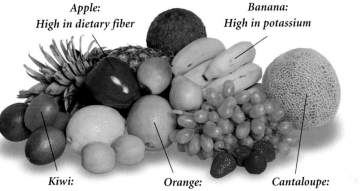

Think Fruit

Apple:
High in dietary fiber

Banana:
High in potassium

Kiwi:
High in magnesium

Orange:
High in calcium

Cantaloupe:
High in Vitamin A

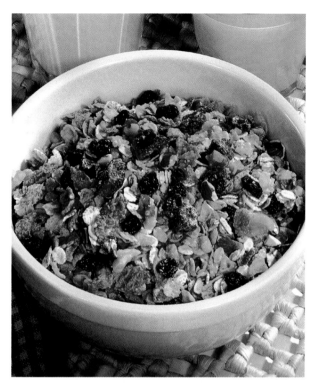

Eating a breakfast balanced with protein, carbohydrates, and fat is a proven way of starting your day alert and lively.

the problem and relaxed diagnostic criteria. Research has consistently absolved sugar from contributing to hyperactivity. More than 20 clinical trials have now looked for such a connection by giving kids meals prepared either with lots of sugar or with artificial sweeteners. Not one found evidence of hyperactivity—in behavior or mental sharpness—after the high-sugar meals. In the trials that included parents' evaluations of their kids, even they couldn't tell the difference.

6. High-carb foods relax some people.

True. In some of the hyperactivity studies, sugary foods slightly relaxed some of the kids. Other evidence suggests that sugar or other high-carb foods—which the body converts to glucose, or simple sugar, in the blood—have a similar effect in adults. One possible explanation: High-carb foods can cause more of the amino acid tryptophan to reach the brain; that in turn can increase the level of serotonin, a nerve chemical that helps control mood.

In many people, however, the apparent ability of carbohydrates to improve mood may do more harm than good. That's because the effect seems to be greatest in people who binge on carbohydrate snacks to make themselves feel better. In such "carbohydrate cravers," the expected mental uplift may encourage unhealthy eating patterns and cause weight gain. "The key is to help those people identify other ways to get that emotional boost," says Bonnie Spring, Ph.D., a researcher at the University of Illinois at Chicago who has studied carbohydrate craving. Exercise can be one effective alternative, says Spring. Bright-light therapy can sometimes help people who also suffer from seasonal affective disorder, or "winter depression," which for unknown reasons often accompanies carb craving.

7. High-carb foods can sharpen the mind.

True (at least in the laboratory). The brain requires glucose to synthesize acetylcholine, which is essential to memory. Since the brain can't store glucose, it needs a constant supply, derived mainly from carbohydrates, to keep functioning at peak capacity. Rats perform better on memory tests after scientists inject glucose directly into their brains. And a number of studies have shown that a pure-glucose drink or high-carbohydrate snack such as a glass of orange juice or a bagel can temporarily boost memory and cognitive performance in humans. However, the benefits were typically quite modest. Moreover, most of those studies were done in people who were fasting. So it's unclear whether consuming additional carbohydrates on top of your regular intake would provide any mental edge—or whether the boost stems from the energy supplied by food in general, not just carbohydrates (see next item).

How well your body regulates blood glucose may affect cognitive function far more than your carbohydrate intake does. Studies show that people who have either a very high or very low glucose level perform worse on a variety of mental tests than people with a normal level. And individuals with diabetes, whose bodies can't regulate blood sugar effectively, are generally more prone than other people to cog-

Orange juice may temporarily boost your memory.

nitive impairment. That provides another reason to try to prevent diabetes, by exercising regularly, losing excess weight, stopping smoking, and consuming plenty of fiber—and for all adults to have their blood-sugar level tested regularly.

8. Eating breakfast can sharpen the mind.

True. Most research—including studies of federally funded school breakfast programs—shows that people who begin the day with breakfast are more alert and lively than those who skip the meal. Moreover, some evidence suggests that any food in the morning can help, not just carbohydrates.

Researchers in Toronto recently gave 22 older volunteers a breakfast drink containing an equal number of calories of either pure carbohydrate, protein, or fat. The carbohydrate drink improved long-term recall for about an hour, compared with 15 minutes for the other drinks. But the protein and fat drinks improved some mental capacities—such as alertness and short-term memory—that the glucose drink didn't.

Another recent study found that a balanced breakfast provides the best overall effect on morning alertness, boosting reaction time, attention span, and memory. Protein and fat not only provide mental benefits complementary to those of carbohydrates but also slow the body's conversion of carbohydrates into blood sugar, providing the brain with a steadier supply of fuel. The bottom line: Don't skip breakfast, and include more than just toast.

9. Eating lunch can sharpen the mind.

True—or false. Whether a midday meal sharpens or dulls your thinking depends on how much you eat. A light lunch or snack can temporarily boost mental acuity, according to a few small studies. But a large lunch, especially one very high in fat or carbohydrates, can increase the sluggishness that normally develops in the early afternoon. (In contrast, a big breakfast does not seem to make people sleepy, perhaps because the natural tendency

*Modest amounts of caffeinated drinks
can help you maintain mental focus.*

toward alertness in the morning obscures that effect.)

10. High-dose caffeine sharpens the mind.

False. Modest amounts of caffeinated drinks—as little as one-third of a cup of brewed coffee—can help people maintain mental focus during monotonous tasks. In one trial, college-age volunteers who drank a cup of coffee beforehand fought off fatigue and absorbed new information better than those who drank decaf.

But large amounts of caffeine can make you jittery and, in turn, impede concentration and memory. Moreover, relying on caffeine as a substitute for sleep when you're trying to learn may be self-defeating. Brain studies in rats show that certain chemical and physical signs of absorbing new information increase during deep sleep. More significant, other research indicates that people retain new material better if they follow the mental workout with either a long nap or a good night's sleep.

SUMMING UP

• The most effective dietary step you can take to protect cognitive function as you age is to eat a diet high in whole grains, produce, and low-fat dairy products. Such a diet, loaded with B vitamins and other beneficial nutrients, will help keep your brain healthy, in part by ensuring that it gets an ample supply of oxygenated blood.

• Eating a well-rounded breakfast, a light lunch, and possibly a snack may help maintain clear thinking throughout the day.

• Whether carbohydrates sharpen the mind better than other foods is not clear. In contrast, they apparently may help some people relax. However, those who binge on carbs for the mood boost should use other methods, such as exercise, instead.

• Caffeine may also boost mental acuity—provided it doesn't make you jittery or unable to sleep.

• Dietary supplements, including ginkgo biloba, probably don't help ward off mental decline or boost cognitive performance. But some—notably St. John's wort and SAM-e—may ease mild emotional problems.

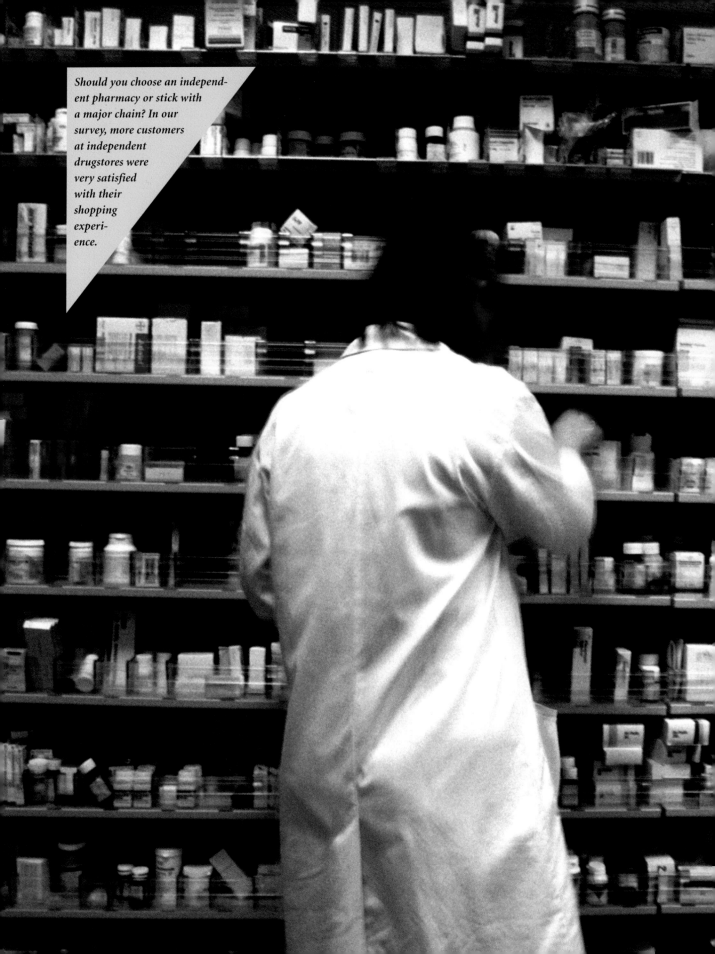

Should you choose an independent pharmacy or stick with a major chain? In our survey, more customers at independent drugstores were very satisfied with their shopping experience.

Time to **switch** drugstores?

I f you're among the 47 percent of Americans who get
medicine from drugstore
giants such as CVS, Eckerd,
and Rite Aid, here's a prescription: Try shopping somewhere
else. The best place to start
looking is one of the 25,000
independent pharmacies that
are making a comeback
throughout the U.S.

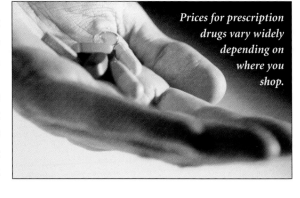

Prices for prescription drugs vary widely depending on where you shop.

Independent stores, which were edging toward extinc-
tion a few years ago, won top honors from CONSUMER
REPORTS readers, besting the big chains by an eye-popping
margin. More than 85 percent of customers at independent drugstores were very satisfied or completely satisfied
with their experience, compared with 58 percent of chain-
drugstore customers.

Many supermarket and mass-merchant pharmacies
also did a better job than the best-known conventional
chains at providing caring, courteous, knowledgeable, and
timely service. And in a nationwide price study we conducted, the chains we evaluated charged the highest
prices—even slightly more than the independents.

Those findings come from our latest investigation into
the best places to shop for prescription medications. More

than 32,000 readers told us
about more than 40,000 experiences at 31 national and
regional drugstore chains (like
CVS, Genovese, Osco, Rite
Aid, and Walgreens); super-
market-pharmacy combos
(such as Kroger, Publix, and
Safeway); mass-merchant
pharmacies (like Costco,
Target, and Wal-Mart); and
independent pharmacies across the nation.

For most consumers, insurance covers at least some of
the cost of prescription drugs, so our Ratings emphasize
service factors that affect everyone. For consumers who
have to pay more than a small percentage of their prescription-drug costs, including more than a third of our
readers, our price study indicated where to save money.
(See "Where to shop, how to save" on page 58.)

Among the other highlights of our research:

• Some of the drugstore chains and supermarkets that
readers favored are family owned or businesses in which
workers have a stake. Medicine Shoppe, the top "chain," is
actually a collection of about 1,000 individually owned
and operated stores with a common parent company.
Among supermarkets, high-rated Wegmans (in New

Jersey, New York, and Pennsylvania) is family owned; and at high-rated Publix (in the South), most workers are stockholders.

• Forty percent of readers said that at least once during the past year, their drugstore was out of the medicine they needed.

• Our market basket of a month's worth of five widely prescribed medications cost $377 to $555, depending on where we shopped. For a family needing all five drugs, that difference would exceed $2,000 a year.

SORTING OUT THE STORES

Most people start by searching for a store that accepts their insurance plan. Fortunately, that isn't the hassle it used to be, especially since independents are accepting more plans these days. Insurers once considered the disparate stores too much trouble to work with, but they realized that keeping independents out of their networks alienated customers and didn't cut costs as much as they'd hoped. Also, 33 states have adopted "any willing provider" laws, which require insurance companies to take into their networks any pharmacy that's willing to accept the insurer's reimbursement rate. As a result, you have a greater choice of where and how to shop. The basic choices:

Independents: Service is all. Prescription drugs are the independents' lifeblood, accounting for 88 percent of sales. That means independents can be a good source of hard-to-find medications. (The chains, where drugs account for 64 percent of sales, tend to focus on the 200 most-prescribed drugs.)

Forty percent of readers said that at least once during the past year, their drugstore was out of the medicine they needed.

That focus on prescriptions can mean more personal attention. Readers said that pharmacists at independent stores were accessible, approachable, and easy to talk to, and that they were especially knowledgeable about medications, both prescription and nonprescription.

The independents (and some chains) offer extras such as disease-management education, in-store health screenings for cholesterol, services such as compounding (customizing medications for patients with special needs), and home delivery.

Many independents are affiliated with programs such as Good Neighbor or Value-Rite, whose names you'll see in the stores. These "banner" programs, offered by wholesale product suppliers, help independents with marketing and with the sale of private-label products, improving purchasing power and name recognition much the way ServiStar and True Value help small hardware stores compete with Home Depot and Lowe's.

About half of the nation's independents have Web sites, where

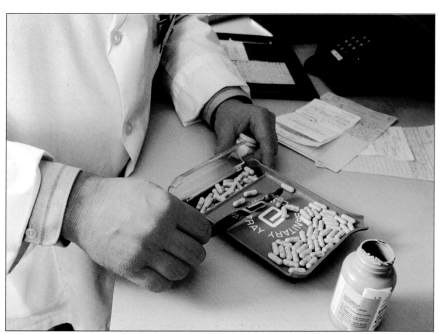

Chains tend to focus on the most-prescribed drugs. Try an independent drugstore for hard-to-find medicines.

The online option: right or risky?

Medications ordered online account for just $3 billion of the $183 billion prescription-drug market. But that figure is expected to quadruple by 2007, according to Jupiter Research. There are time- and money-saving reasons for trying a Web site, but you'll need to proceed with care, especially if the site isn't affiliated with a brick-and-mortar store. Here are some basic guidelines:

When to go online. Web pharmacies have the edge for medications that manage chronic conditions, for which you need less advice from the druggist. And they're the choice when you need a large supply. Online, you may be able to order three- to six-months' worth, depending on insurance coverage.

When not to. If you need medicine in a hurry, unaffiliated online pharmacies aren't the answer unless you're willing to pay the extra $15 or so for overnight delivery. They are also inappropriate for certain narcotics (for instance, some medicines containing codeine). Many state and federal laws limit shipment of such drugs.

Ill-legit? Many sites peddle drugs for weight loss,

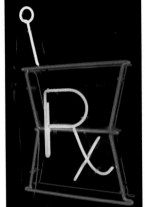

baldness, you name it—yet require no doctor's visit for a prescription. Increasingly, they are pitching stronger drugs, such as anabolic steroids.

Choosing the right site. Any legitimate online drugstore will require a prescription, meet government regulations, and have a license to fill prescriptions in every state where it does business. The National Association of Boards of Pharmacy has developed a voluntary program dubbed VIPPS, for Verified Internet Pharmacy Practice Site, to help consumers identify companies that are licensed by and in good standing with regulatory agencies. Approved sites display the VIPPS seal.

The program is voluntary and doesn't list all legitimate operators. If you plan to buy from an unfamiliar site, make sure it has a verifiable phone number and address (not a P.O. box), and that it identifies the the presiding pharmacist or practitioner. You can check whether any site is licensed by a state pharmacy board by visiting *www.nabp.net*. Make sure the site's privacy policy is clearly stated and promises not to divulge personal information unless legally required.

---

you can generally order medicine and find some health information but not much more.

Chains: Convenient but crowded. With about 20,000 stores nationwide, mega-drugstores are in nearly everyone's backyard. Many are open around the clock, have a drive-through pharmacy for faster pickup, and let you order online or by punching a few numbers on a telephone. You can even set up your Web account to have renewals automatically processed and readied for pickup or mailing. The biggest chains let you check prices online. Another advantage: The chains accept payment from lots of health plans (managed care pays for 80 percent of all conventional-chain prescriptions).

Now for the drawbacks. The chains' locations in populous areas and their acceptance of a plethora of plans has made them, in effect, too popular, and service is suffering. Except for Medicine Shoppe, chains typically made readers wait longer, were slower to fill orders, and provided less personal attention than other types of drugstores.

Like other drugstores, the chains have experienced shrinking reimbursement from insurers. They've helped maintain profits by selling everything from milk to Halloween costumes. That makes one-stop shopping possible (if your list isn't too specific), but it also can create bottlenecks at the checkout.

Supermarkets: One stop does it. There are fewer than 9,000 supermarkets that include a pharmacy, but the number is rising. One-stop shopping is the attraction. Many supermarkets put the pharmacy near the entrance for easy access and to attract store traffic. For those very reasons, however, you may not have as much privacy to consult with the druggist as you would elsewhere.

Supermarkets have online pharmacy sites, usually as a link from the home page, but they're often less comprehensive than those of big drugstore chains.

Mass merchants: Low price is key. Like supermarkets,

Where to shop, how to save

You can cut bills substantially by comparison shopping, as we discovered in a price study at 130 pharmacies of five drugs: Celebrex, Lipitor, Norvasc, Prevacid, and Zoloft. Online pharmacies and mass merchants delivered the lowest prices overall, trailed by supermarkets, independents, and drug chains. That was true even when we factored in standard shipping for the Web sites. Exceptions to the "online is cheap" rule: *www.clickpharmacy.com* and *www.cvs.com*, where prices were higher than at all three of the mass merchants we studied.

Among the online places with the best prices were *www.familymeds.com*, which also operates more than 100 brick-and-mortar stores in 16 states; *www.costco.com* (the store charges $45 a year for membership, but no membership is required to order from the Web site); and *www.drugstore.com*, a Web site with no stores.

At the least expensive individual store of all, our market basket cost $377; at the most expensive, $555. Prices from one independent to the next varied, of course, but so did prices among stores within other categories. Perhaps most surprising was the inconsistency in stores within the very same chain. At a Safeway in Chicago, the blood-pressure drug Norvasc cost $76; at a Safeway in Las Vegas, it cost $43.

Do your homework. Sites such as *www.pillbot.com* (free) and *www.pharmacychecker.com* (usually $25 per year) can help you compare prices. Other tips:

Ask for generics. They usually cost 25 to 50 percent less than brand-name equivalents. Keep in mind that when a new generic drug hits the market, it may be only slightly cheaper, but the cost drops further as other generics are approved.

Buy in bulk. If you're taking medication for a chronic condition, ask your doctor if the prescription can cover more than the standard 30 days, which could reduce the cost per pill. If insurance is paying, there may be a time or dose limit; self-payers have more control. You can generally buy greater quantities online.

Seek a senior discount. Many stores offer 10 percent off if you're 65 or older.

Check your drugstore's Web site. Medicine may cost more at the store than on the Web. The average price difference between Eckerd and Walgreens stores and sites, for example, varied by about 15 percent. To get the Web price, you can't pick up your order; it must be mailed.

The bottom line for five top drugs

Average total cost reflects prices for a 30-day supply of five drugs from 130 individual merchants (8 Web sites plus 12 stores each for most of the mass merchants, supermarkets, and chains and 15 for the independents). For Web sites, shipping costs are in parentheses.

Outlet	Average total cost
ONLINE	**$412**
www.familymeds.com	377 (free shipping)
www.costco.com	395 (free)
www.drugstore.com	398 ($1.49)
www.eckerd.com	408 ($3.95; free over $40)
www.walgreens.com	415 ($1.95)
www.aarppharmacy.com	420 ($2.25)
www.clickpharmacy.com	429 ($6.95; free over $65)
www.cvs.com	454 ($1.95)
MASS MERCHANTS	**$416**
Costco	399
Target	421
Wal-Mart	425
SUPERMARKETS	**$464**
Albertsons	454
Safeway	460
Kroger	479
INDEPENDENTS	**$470**
DRUG CHAINS	**$481**
CVS	478
Eckerd	481
Walgreens	484

(Chart originally appeared in the October 2003 issue of CONSUMER REPORTS.)

Think twice about discount cards. One study concluded that a single card is unlikely to suit everyone. A spokeswoman at the General Accounting Office, which conducted its own study, suggested that consumers might save as much on their own if they work at it. We agree. When our reporter presented the ProCare Card ($5 to enroll and $15.95 a month for family coverage) at a local Walgreens, the price for our market basket was $73 less than the chain's national average—but only $4 less than what we would have paid, without a card, at *www.walgreens.com*. The Member Rx card from AARP ($19.95 a year) shaved just $19 off AARP's prices for our market basket. At Costco, Target, and *www.drugstore.com*, we saved more than with either card.

these stores sell a wide variety of goods. But their main draw is low prices. One in five readers who bought medication from a mass merchant had no prescription-drug coverage. In our price study, only Web sites sold medications as cheaply. In our survey, ShopKo and Target were among the high-rated mass merchants; Wal-Mart was worse than most others.

All of the mass merchants in our survey have Web sites for ordering prescriptions, but only the Costco site lets you check drug prices.

Online: Low prices, no face time. Virtual pharmacies come in two basic flavors. There are adjuncts to brick-and-mortar stores, where you can order online and receive your prescription by mail or pick it up. Then there are sites such as *www.drugstore.com* and *www.aarppharmacy.com*, which have no store and simply mail the medicine to you. With both types of site, you can enter the name and quantity of the drug online; a pharmacist will confirm the prescription with your doctor. (Often, you can fax or mail a paper prescription instead and wait for it to be approved, but that can add days to the process.)

Anytime you're not picking up from a pharmacist, you lose a chance for personal contact, a consideration if you're using a medication for the first time or are juggling medications. To compensate, the stand-alone Web sites—and those operated by the drug chains and some mass merchants—make it easy to e-mail questions to pharmacists 24/7, research medical topics, search online for potentially dangerous drug interactions, receive e-mail refill reminders, keep track of your medications, and note any drug allergies. Drugstore.com will also alert you if the branded drug you're taking becomes available in generic form.

It can take as little as a couple of hours for your medicine to be ready if you order from a chain and are willing to retrieve it, or as long as three to five business days if you ask for it to be mailed standard shipping. That's free or nearly so. You can pay about $15 to have medicine overnighted (refrigerated medicines must be sent that

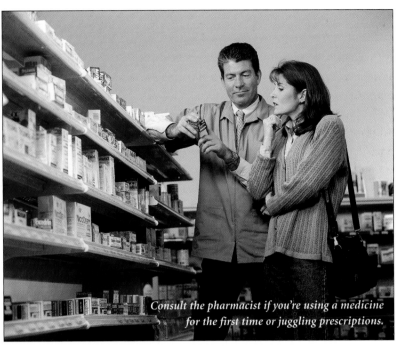

Consult the pharmacist if you're using a medicine for the first time or juggling prescriptions.

way). Web sites can't ship every controlled substance.

When you use a Web site, you can avoid waiting in line, of course, and you'll tend to pay lower prices, even when shipping costs are included. No computer? No problem. Sites have toll-free numbers.

Four percent of our readers had bought medications online, most often from drug chains, and three-quarters of those said the transaction went smoothly: Their order was processed quickly enough for their needs, and e-mailed questions were answered promptly. (For details on ordering via the Web, see "The online option" on page 57.)

GETTING BETTER SERVICE

Some stores did far better than others in service, speed, and information provided by the druggist. The most frequent complaints: Drugs were out of stock, readers had to wait a long time for service at the pharmacy counter, and prescriptions weren't ready.

Drugstore chains and supermarkets were most likely to be out of a requested drug. When a drug was out of stock, independents were able to obtain it within one day 80 percent of the time, vs. about 55 to 60 percent for the other types of stores. Only 9 percent of the time did independent customers have to wait at least three days for an out-of-stock drug or find it elsewhere, vs. at least 18 percent of the time for other types of stores.

Drugs were out of stock more often this time than when we published our last drugstore survey, in 1999. The steepest jump took place at Albertsons, Giant, and Longs Drugs, whose out-of-stocks increased by more than 15 percentage points. That's probably the case in part because the number of prescriptions being written is growing faster than the shelf space.

Overall, 27 percent of readers complained about long waits. It's no wonder. Pharmacists fill nearly 4 billion prescriptions a year, an average of almost 200 per day for each pharmacist, and spend one-fourth of their time on

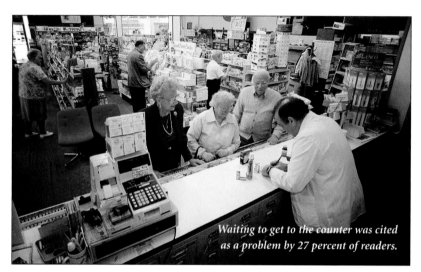
Waiting to get to the counter was cited as a problem by 27 percent of readers.

administrative work such as calling doctors and dealing with insurance companies. Moreover, there's a shortage of druggists—there are approximately 5,500 job openings around the U.S. At CVS, Genovese, Longs Drugs, and Sav-On, about 40 percent of readers complained of long waits for service. Lines were short at Medicine Shoppe (only 6 percent of readers complained) and at the independents (8 percent).

Twenty percent of readers overall said that their prescription wasn't ready when promised. Among the worst offenders: CVS, Genovese, and Rite Aid, where prescriptions weren't ready nearly one-third of the time. Better-prepared stores included Medicine Shoppe, Publix, ShopKo, Winn-Dixie, and the independents.

Other complaints focused on how pharmacists interact with customers. Worst offenders: the drugstore chains, where 10 percent of readers said they did not receive enough personal attention from their pharmacist. Best:

You guessed it —the independents—where only 2 percent of readers found fault.

Service may improve in all stores, eventually. In many states, regulators are giving technicians more authority to assist druggists. Technology is also lending a hand in the form of robotic machines that dispense medications. They do everything but cap the bottle (which goes uncapped to the pharmacist for a final inspection).

Although only a small fraction of doctors are now writing e-prescriptions, they are the wave of the future. Doctors use a handheld device to transmit your prescription to the drugstore. The procedure avoids one of druggists' biggest problems and a contributor to the rising incidence of drug errors: deciphering doctors' handwriting.

While waiting for the future, you might improve the odds of getting good service now by patronizing an independent pharmacy. But whatever drugstore you use, you're apt to get better service by following some simple advice:

Avoid waiting. Order drugs online or by phone, then pick them up (or, if you're not in a rush, have them mailed). If you plan to pick up drugs, check from home whether the doctor and druggist have connected and the prescription is ready.

Establish a good relationship. Make sure you can step aside and talk privately with the pharmacist and that you can reach him or her by phone. The pharmacist should volunteer details about the drug and be able to answer questions about nonprescription products, too. With online pharmacies, make sure you receive prompt, thorough answers to questions submitted by e-mail.

Get good advice. Check that the pharmacy keeps and updates your medication records, which should reduce the risk of a drug conflict or adverse reaction. Don't walk away from the counter without knowing the following: what to do if you miss a dose; how many refills are permitted; how to store the drug and when it expires; what side effects to expect, along with which to ignore and which to contact your doctor about; and foods, drugs, supplements, or situations to avoid while taking the medication.

Going off-label with drugs

A label on a prescription drug is a lot more than the little sticker that comes on the bottle you get from the pharmacy. It is an FDA-approved document, typically running to several pages of blindingly minuscule type, covering the drug's chemical makeup, effectiveness, dosage range, the reasons for prescribing it, side effects, and any other material the FDA deems important.

The relevant label information for the typical patient includes the disorder that the FDA approved the drug for, based on the results of clinical trials. If a drug is prescribed for that reason, it is called an on-label use. Any deviation from the label is deemed an off-label use.

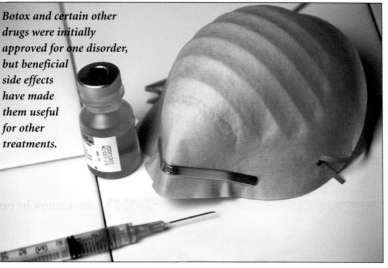

Botox and certain other drugs were initially approved for one disorder, but beneficial side effects have made them useful for other treatments.

Once a drug has been approved, physicians can use that drug for any purpose that they believe represents "reasonable and current" prescribing practices, whether or not it's on the label.

How do off-label indications come to be? Often they arise from side effects that crop up during therapy for the FDA-approved indication. For instance, an occasional side effect of spironolactone (Aldactone), a mild diuretic used for the treatment of hypertension, is enlargement of the male breast. The ability of this drug to mimic a female hormone led to successful treatment of women with unwanted, excess hair.

Similar unexpected observations led to the use of botulinum toxin (Botox) injections—originally approved for facial wrinkles—for severe, intractable migraine headaches. Other examples, among hundreds, include the use of topiramate (Topamax), an antiseizure drug, to treat chronic-pain syndromes, and terazosin (Hytrin), a blood-pressure drug, for enlarged prostates. Many of the multidrug chemotherapy protocols for cancer treatment represent off-label drug use.

Off-label drug use is only as good as the evidence on which it is based. And that can vary from a randomized placebo-controlled study in a peer-reviewed medical journal all the way down to an anecdotal case report—or, even worse, a hunch, guesswork, or successful overpromotion of the drug to doctors by the manufacturer. But reimbursement and legal considerations make most physicians fairly cautious about prescribing off-label without a good reason.

Once a drug is being used widely off-label, there is little financial incentive for its manufacturer to apply to the FDA to legitimize that use by putting it on the label. The required clinical trials are expensive, and there's always the risk that the FDA will turn down the additional indication.

GETTING INFORMATION

Unbiased consumer and physician information about valid off-label drug use is not easy to find. *The Physicians' Desk Reference* includes only approved drug indications. The *2005 Consumer Drug Reference*, published by CONSUMER REPORTS (available at *www.ConsumerReports.org* or at 800-500-9760),

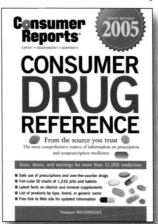

has some information on off-label uses provided by experts from the United States Pharmacopeia. There is also information available online, but be sure it comes from a trustworthy source, such as a university medical center. Avoid commercial sources.

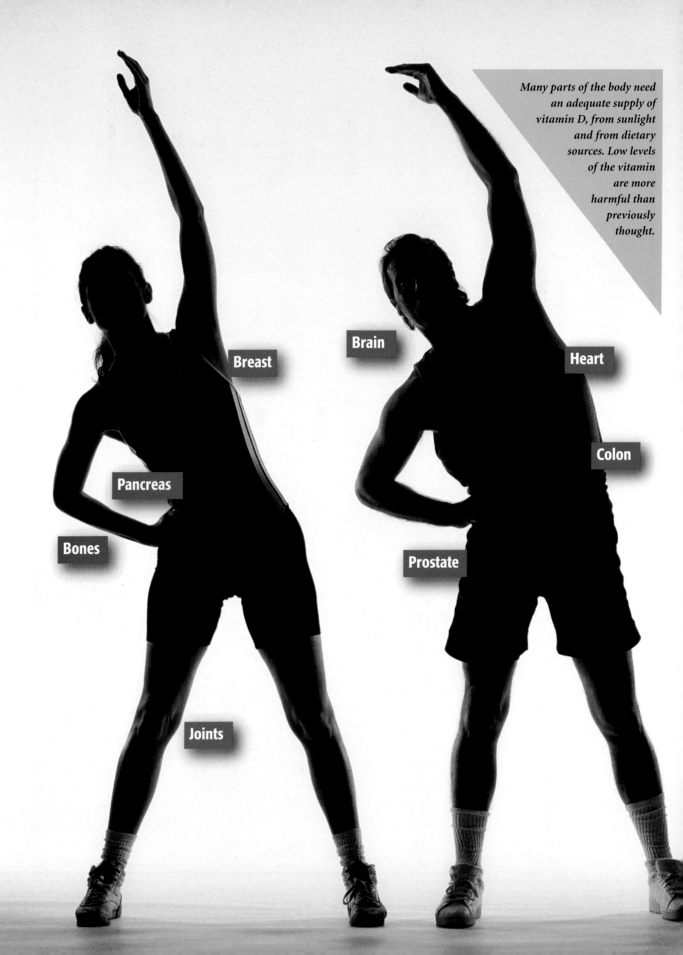

Many parts of the body need an adequate supply of vitamin D, from sunlight and from dietary sources. Low levels of the vitamin are more harmful than previously thought.

Breast

Brain

Heart

Colon

Pancreas

Prostate

Bones

Joints

Do you need more Vitamin D?

When the shorter, darker days of winter loom, we all miss the sun's warming rays. Our bodies also miss the sunshine vitamin—vitamin D—if we haven't stored enough of it during the spring, summer, and fall. Research has shown that insufficient levels of vitamin D are far more common and far more harmful than previously believed.

While too much sunlight can cause skin cancer, one study estimates that tens of thousands of Americans die each year of cancers possibly caused by too little sun exposure and, in turn, too little vitamin D. (The average person gets about 90 percent of the vitamin from sunlight, the rest from dietary sources.) Moreover, shortfalls of sun and vitamin D may weaken the bones, possibly worsen arthritis, and perhaps increase the risk of heart disease, diabetes, and other disorders.

Low vitamin-D levels are surprisingly common, especially during northern winters. In one study, nearly one-third of Bostonians had inadequate stores of the vitamin at the end of the cold months, compared with only 4 percent at summer's end. Other research shows that people who are older, black, or overweight face the highest risk of having too little D.

This report will help you determine whether you need to get more vitamin D—and how to get it safely if you do.

THE RISKS OF TOO LITTLE D

Here are the most significant hazards of getting insufficient amounts of the vitamin:

• **Weak bones, aching joints.** Vitamin D helps the body absorb calcium from food, thereby making more of the mineral available to the bones. Outright deficiency of the vitamin prevents new bone tissue from hardening, a condition known as rickets in children, osteomalacia in adults. And vitamin-D deficiency clearly worsens osteoporosis, the brittle-bone disease.

Got vitamin D? Vitamin-D fortified milk may help the body absorb calcium for strong bones.

But even moderately low levels of vitamin D, traditionally considered within the normal range, may also weaken the bones and increase the risk of fractures. Such moderate declines in the vitamin cause the body to churn out extra parathyroid hormone, which tends to pull calcium out of the skeleton. Studies show that consuming more vitamin D by itself can slow bone loss and possibly

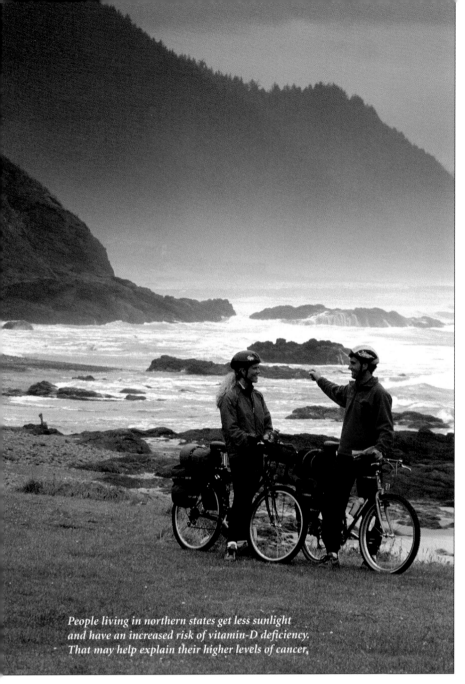

People living in northern states get less sunlight and have an increased risk of vitamin-D deficiency. That may help explain their higher levels of cancer.

• **Cancer.** Researchers have long known that cancer-death rates in the U.S. are higher in the North than in the South, but they've failed to identify any dietary or lifestyle factor to explain why. William Grant, Ph.D., an atmospheric scientist who investigates connections between the environment and health, has compared cancer mortality in various parts of the country

In overweight people, vitamin D gets trapped in fat cells, which can create deficiencies.

that receive different amounts of sunlight. Reduced sunlight correlated with increased risk for 13 types of cancer, notably of the breast, colon, ovary, and prostate, as well as non-Hodgkins lymphoma. Grant estimates that, if those correlations represent a true causal connection, nearly 24,000 Americans per year are dying from cancers caused by insufficient sunlight. Grant's findings support the results of several previous studies that also found reduced cancer rates in sunny regions, both here and abroad.

To explain that connection, Grant and other scientists point to research linking low vitamin-D levels with increased risk of both colon cancer and prostate cancer. Moreover, vitamin D inhibits the development and growth of various cancers in animals. In fact, some cancer specialists are now testing vitamin D as a treatment for prostate and colon cancer.

• **Heart disease.** People with thin bones often have extensive calcium deposits in their arteries. Researchers theorize that the parathyroid-hormone buildup sparked by vitamin-D insufficiency may not only leach calcium

increase bone density in older women who have low-normal levels of the vitamin. Boosting the intake of both vitamin D and calcium can reduce the risk of fracture—and may help prevent tooth loss—in those women.

Finally, vitamin D may possibly slow the progression of osteoarthritis, the most common type of joint inflammation. In one test of that theory, Boston researchers studied 75 arthritic knees for up to 10 years. The disease was three times as likely to become worse in people who had average or lower vitamin-D levels as in those who had higher levels of the vitamin.

out of the bones but also dump it in the arteries, contributing to the development of vessel-clogging plaque deposits. Moreover, parathyroid-hormone elevations may possibly raise blood pressure, further increasing coronary risk. A few studies have indeed linked low vitamin-D levels with increased likelihood of both calcified arteries and coronary disease. For example, an 11-year observational study of some 10,000 women in California found that those who took vitamin-D supplements were one-third less likely than others to die of coronary disease.

• **Diabetes.** The pancreas needs vitamin D to produce the hormone insulin, which controls blood-sugar levels. Lack of the vitamin appears to increase the risk of type 1 (insulin-dependent) diabetes, the less common but more serious type. People in the higher, darker latitudes face an increased risk of type 1, and they tend to develop it at a younger age. Three large studies have found lower rates of the disease in children who received vitamin-D supplements as infants or whose mothers took the supplements during pregnancy.

• **Schizophrenia and multiple sclerosis.** Vitamin D stimulates production of certain nerve or brain chemicals that may help prevent schizophrenia and multiple sclerosis (MS). Both conditions arise more often in populations that get little sunlight. And vitamin D has reversed MS in mice.

WHO'S AT RISK

While researchers have not yet determined exactly how much vitamin D the body needs, many experts lean toward a blood level of at least 20 nanograms per milliliter; that's the amount required to keep the parathyroid-hormone blood level down.

Young and middle-aged white people in sunny regions, including the American South, almost always get that much vitamin D from sunshine alone, just by going about their daily affairs. But almost everyone else is at risk for vitamin-D insufficiency, especially in the winter. Numerous studies have found substantial wintertime drops in vitamin-D levels. Indeed, average bone density falls and fracture risk rises in winter, the latter caused only

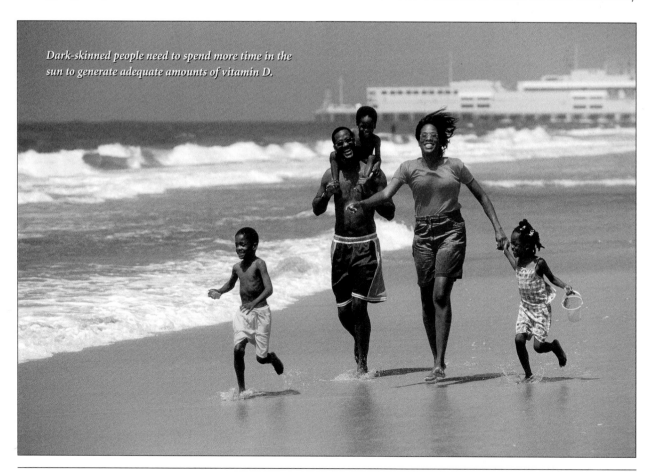

Dark-skinned people need to spend more time in the sun to generate adequate amounts of vitamin D.

Vitamin D in the diet

Listed at right are the most common sources of vitamin D in the diet. Three of them—seafood, mushrooms, and eggs—are the only foods that naturally contain the vitamin. The fourth source, milk, is routinely fortified with D. (The vitamin may also be added to other foods, including breads, breakfast cereals, fruit drinks, chocolate beverages, and cocoa powder; check the label to see.)

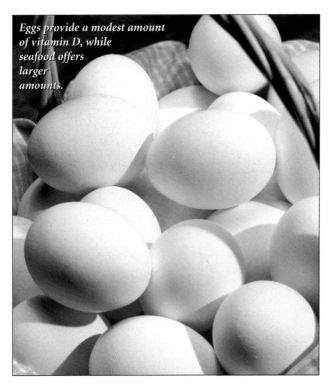

Eggs provide a modest amount of vitamin D, while seafood offers larger amounts.

Food	Serving size	Vitamin D (IU)
DAIRY		
Milk*	1 cup	100**
Egg, whole	1	26
FISH AND SHELLFISH		
Oysters	3 oz	544
Cod-liver oil	1 tsp	452
Catfish	3 oz	424
Mackerel	3 oz	394
Salmon	3 oz	238
Sardines, canned in oil	3 oz	231
Tuna, bluefin	3 oz	170
Halibut	3 oz	170
Tuna, canned in water	3 oz	136
Shrimp	3 oz	122
Sole/flounder	3 oz	51
Cod	3 oz	48
Bass, freshwater	3 oz	34
Swordfish	3 oz	34
Clams	3 oz	7
MUSHROOMS		
Shitake	2 oz	57
Chanterelle	2 oz	48

IU = International Units * Whole, reduced-fat, low-fat, or non-fat milk.
** While each cup of milk is supposed to be fortified with 100 IU of vitamin D, studies have not yet proved the reliability of the fortification process. Chart originally appeared in the November 2004 issue of CONSUMER REPORTS on Health newsletter .

partly by slips on ice and snow. In addition to winter and living in dark, high-latitude regions, the following factors also increase the chance of vitamin-D insufficiency:

• **Older age.** Studies have repeatedly shown that most people over age 65 or so have insufficient vitamin-D levels, for several reasons. They tend to wear protective clothing, apply strong sunscreens, and stay indoors more often than younger people. Their skin's ability to synthesize the vitamin is reduced. (Lengthier sun exposure doesn't help; instead, older people need to compensate by exposing more skin, as described later in this article.) And they're more likely to take certain drugs, notably laxatives and the cholesterol-lowering drug cholestyramine (Questran), that interfere with the absorption of the vitamin.

• **Darker skin color.** The darker your skin, the more sunlight you need to generate vitamin D. Researchers from the Centers for Disease Control and Prevention recently concluded that on average some 40 percent of black women were low in the vitamin. In theory, says Michael F. Holick, Ph.D., M.D., a vitamin-D expert at Boston University Medical Center, the rates in black men should be roughly the same.

• **Excess weight.** Vitamin D is fat soluble. So in overweight individuals, substantial amounts of the vitamin manufactured by the skin get trapped in the excess fat cells. As a result, obese individuals on average have about two-thirds less vitamin D in their blood than other people and are thus typically deficient in the vitamin.

THE VITAMIN-D PRESCRIPTION

Judicious sun exposure can provide most people with all the vitamin D they need. The best time of day is mid-morning or midafternoon—earlier or later than that during summer in the South—when the sun is typically neither too strong to damage the skin easily nor too weak to stimulate vitamin-D production. To obtain enough vitamin D for the entire year, seek sun exposure during three seasons: spring, summer, and fall in the North (because there the winter sun is too weak to stimulate vitamin production), and any three seasons in the South.

Regardless of their race, people who are overweight or older than age 60 or so should expose their hands and lower arms as well as their face or lower legs without sunscreen about three times a week for roughly one-quarter the time it takes their skin to start turning red. People who are younger or thinner need to expose only their hands and lower arms. During the optimal hours in June, it typically takes about 40 minutes for the skin to start to redden in white people living anywhere in a rough line linking Boston, Chicago, and southern Oregon—so they'd need about 10 minutes of daily exposure. Darker skin increases that time by up to 50 percent; it also increases with higher latitudes and in months before or after June. Conversely, the time decreases with lighter skin and lower latitudes.

People who can't or won't spend the necessary time outdoors need to consider dietary sources of the vitamin. Our medical consultants say that middle-aged and

Older people need higher amounts of vitamin D, ideally from sunshine.

The table on the facing page lists foods rich in vitamin D. If you don't consume enough of those foods to reach the recommended dietary intake for your age and sun-exposure level, consider taking a supplement.

That's particularly appropriate in winter and among people at increased risk for osteoporosis. Risk factors include being a postmenopausal woman, especially one whose menopause started early or who consumed little calcium as a child or premenopausal woman; family history of osteoporosis; lack of weight-bearing exercise; heavy alcohol intake; smoking cigarettes; and being thin, white, or Asian.

If you do take a vitamin-D supplement, be sure it contains no more than the dose that brings you up to roughly the amount described above for your age group. The typical multivitamin contains 400 IU of vitamin D—enough for young or middle-aged people exposed to some

People who can't or are unable to spend the necessary time outdoors need to consider dietary sources of the vitamin.

younger people who get some but not enough sunshine need about 400 International Units (IU) of vitamin D per day; older persons need 600 to 800 IU. People of any age who rarely or never get out in the sun probably need about 1,000 IU.

However, obtaining even the lower amount of vitamin D from food can be difficult. Few foods other than fatty fish are good natural sources of the vitamin, and the most common fortified food is milk, which many people avoid.

but not enough sun and for similarly exposed older people who regularly consume lots of milk or fish; other persons may need a higher-dose supplement, containing 600 to 1,000 IU. However, too much vitamin D (more than about 2,000 IU per day) can lead to elevated calcium levels and, in turn, kidney damage and calcium deposits throughout the body. But it's impossible to get a toxic dose of vitamin D from sun exposure; that's a self-regulating mechanism.

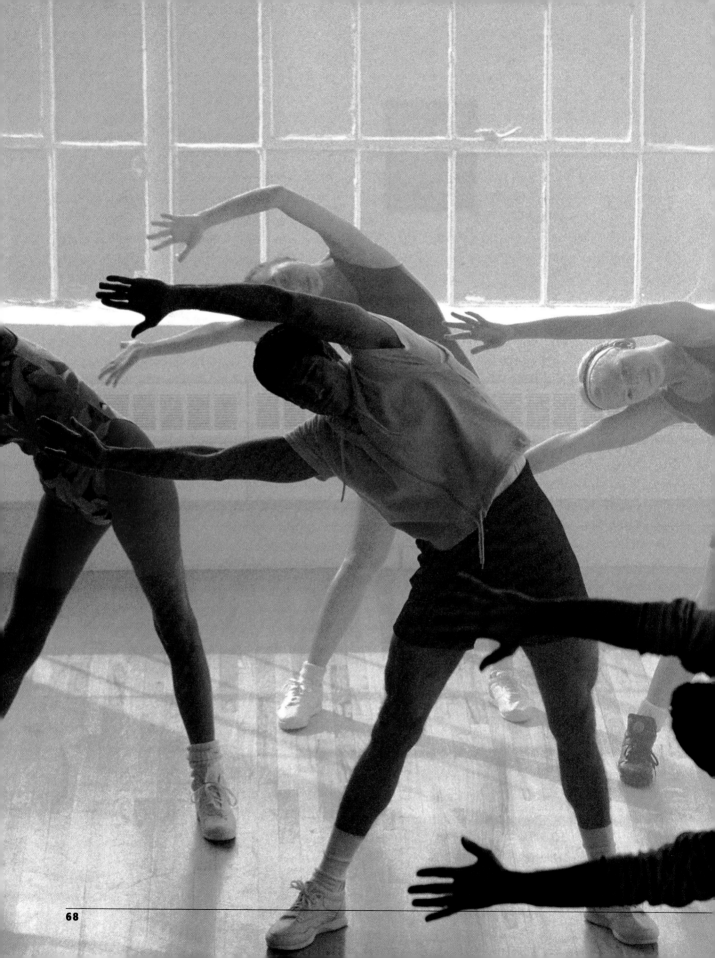

Fitness & Exercise

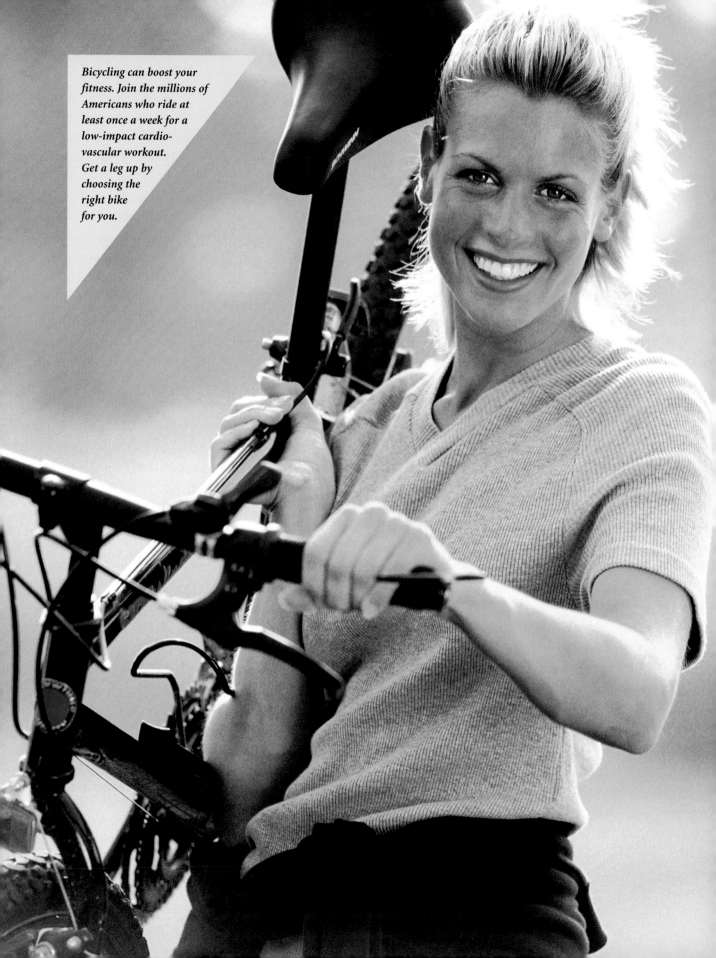

Bicycling can boost your fitness. Join the millions of Americans who ride at least once a week for a low-impact cardio-vascular workout. Get a leg up by choosing the right bike for you.

More bike for the buck

If you plan to buy one of the 19 million new bikes Americans will pedal home this year, chances are your new ride will have an aluminum frame, even if it costs less than $500. It might even have disc brakes or 27 gears. These features, once found only on more expensive bikes, bring the benefits of lighter weight, better braking in sloppy conditions, and more efficient pedaling to cyclists with a modest budget.

Higher-priced bikes are getting better, too. The best of the $1,000-and-up models we tested had the shock absorption and handling previously found only on bikes costing two or three times as much.

For this report, we tested four types of bikes representing the majority of all adult bikes sold: full-suspension mountain bikes, front-suspension mountain bikes, hybrids, and comfort bikes. Prices for the 24 bikes in the "Ratings" chart ranged from $280 to $1,450. (In 2003 we tested road bikes for high-speed or high-mileage rides. See "Get the right bike for the road," on page 72, for recommendations based on those tests.)

Whichever bike you choose, there's good reason to buy it from one of the nation's 5,300 bike shops, rather than from a department or toy store. And you don't have to spend a fortune. We found fine choices for pavement rides that cost less than $300 and very good bikes for off-road cycling for $440. The bikes for serious trail riding cost $1,000 or more, and they're worth every penny.

HOW TO CHOOSE

Decide where you'll ride. Each type of bike is designed for a different kind of terrain and use. The "Types" section (page 73) can help you find a bike that's best for the kind of riding you prefer, whether that's off-road or on, punishing trail or inviting path, serious mileage or brief jaunt.

Focus on fit. It's important to get a bike frame that's the right size. To make sure a frame isn't too tall or short, straddle the bike and measure the clearance between your crotch and the top tube. Depending on the design, there should be 1 to 3 inches of space for hybrid and comfort bikes, 3 to 6 inches for mountain bikes. Handlebars should be at a comfortable height and reach. Have a pro help you get the best fit and feel by adjusting or changing components like the handlebar stem, saddle, seatpost, or cranks.

Deal with a bike shop. You'll generally pay $250 or more at a bike shop, versus $100 and up in a department or discount store, but you'll get more for the money. The bikes tend to be better-made, and you can usually road test them. Most come in several sizes, often including versions proportioned for women. (Women with a longer-than-average torso may get a better fit with a "man's" frame.) Some women's bikes have a step-through frame, but others have the same standard frame as men's bikes. The staff typically knows how to fit you for a frame and adjust components. Bike-shop mechanics tend to do a better job assembling bikes than department-store employees, and bike shops offer after-sale service. A shop can help you choose a helmet, too (see page 77).

Don't be cheap. A bargain price sounds enticing, but you get what you pay for. Bikes selling for $100 to $200 are usually heavier than higher-priced bikes, harder to pedal and shift, and unlikely to fit well because most come in only one frame size. When we tested three mass-market bikes, their quality and performance were below those of the bikes in the "Ratings." (See "Cheap Bikes are not Bargains" on page 76.) Consider low-priced bikes only for the most casual adult riders or for kids who will quickly outgrow them.

Customize components.
Handlebars, handlebar stems, seatposts, saddles, and pedals come in various configurations. (See "Features" chart on page 75.)

Treat it right.
Take your new bike back to the shop to get it adjusted after riding it for a month or so. Keep the gears and chain clean. Have a pro tune up the bike once a year to keep the gear train, brakes, bearings, and suspension working well and to prevent premature wear from dirt, rust, and loose components.

Get the right bike for the road.
For fast or long rides on pavement, consider a road bike. Lighter than other bikes, these have thin tires and other features for distance use. Of the road bikes we tested last year, three good ones are still available and haven't changed significantly: the Trek 1200, $850; the Raleigh Grand Prix, $880; and the Cannondale R400 Triple, $800.

Quick Picks

With a few exceptions, the bikes within each group had their own personalities but offered similar overall performance and pricing. Highlighted are models you might want to consider based on how they scored and on price and features. (Numbers refer to Ratings, p.76)

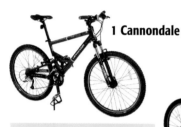

1 Cannondale

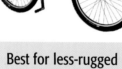

6 Gary Fisher

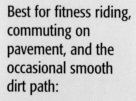

14 Giant

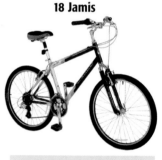

18 Jamis

Best for rough, hilly terrain:

1 Cannondale $1,100
2 Specialized $1,200
3 Trek $1,150
4 Giant $1,450

Of these full-suspension bikes, the Cannondale (1) had the softest ride and is best if you prefer plush downhill shock absorption to riding efficiency. The Specialized (2) had the best blend of downhill shock absorption and efficiency. The Trek (3) and Giant (4) sacrificed some plushness for efficiency on smooth terrain and climbs. While pricey, the Giant is the lightest.

Best for less-rugged off-road trails:

6 Gary Fisher $450
7 Specialized $440
8 Trek $440
9 Raleigh $450

These front-suspension models cost much less than full-suspension bikes but still provide adequate shock absorption for moderate off-road riding. They're also more efficient for pedaling on roads. The Specialized (7) was smoothest of this group.

Best for fitness riding, commuting on pavement, and the occasional smooth dirt path:

14 Giant $470
15 Jamis $480
16 Gary Fisher $470

With larger wheels, narrower tires, and a lighter frame than mountain bikes, these hybrids are better for moderate speeds on pavement than for rough-and-ready off-road riding. The Giant (14) and Jamis (15) stressed smoothness; the Gary Fisher (16) an aggressive, fitness-oriented ride.

Best for casual cycling on pavement and the occasional smooth dirt path:

18 Jamis $300
19 GT $300
20 Trek $300
21 Schwinn $300

A sturdy frame, wide tires, and shock-absorbing fork and seatpost make these comfort bikes perfect for neighborhood rides. All have twist-type shifters; all but the Jamis (18) have high-rise handlebars.

Types Choose a bike that's best suited to the kind of riding you do.

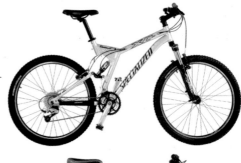

For rough terrain with steep slopes

Best choice: Full-suspension mountain bike ————————
What you'll get: A shock-absorbing suspension fork and rear-suspension frame, which provide the best control and comfort on the roughest terrain. Most have 27 speeds and 26-inch wheels. All have wide, knobby tires; narrow or moderate-width saddle; and flat or riser handlebars.
Expect to pay: $1,000 to more than $4,000.

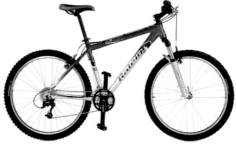

For less-rugged off-road trails

Best choice: Front-suspension mountain bike ————————
What you'll get: A shock-absorbing suspension fork and rigid frame, fine for tamer trails. These bikes need less maintenance and are more efficient on smooth terrain. Most have 24 or 27 speeds; 26-inch wheels; wide, knobby tires; narrow or moderately wide saddle; and flat or riser handlebars.
Expect to pay: $400 to more than $2,000.

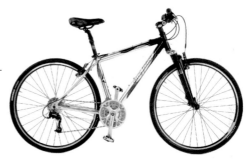

For moderate-speed riding on pavement and smooth dirt paths

Best choice: Hybrid bike ————————
What you'll get: A cross between comfort and road bikes, most have a shock-absorbing suspension fork and seatpost; 24 speeds; 700C wheels (a designation from the French system, indicating size and width; it's about 27-inch); midwidth, fairly smooth tires; moderately wide saddle; and riser handlebars.
Expect to pay: $400 to more than $500.

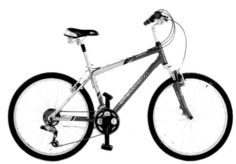

For casual cycling on pavement and smooth dirt paths

Best choice: Comfort bike ————————
What you'll get: Most have a shock-absorbing suspension fork and seatpost; 21 speeds; 26-inch wheels; wide, relatively smooth tires; wide saddle; and riser handlebars. Generally have most upright riding position, which casual riders often find most comfortable.
Expect to pay: $250 to more than $400.

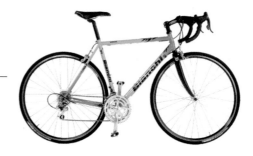

For fast and/or long-distance rides on pavement

Best choice: Road bike ————————
What you'll get: Most have a lightweight frame with no suspension; 18 to 30 speeds; 700C wheels (about 27-inch); narrow, smooth tires; narrow saddle; and drop handlebars. The bent-over riding position reduces wind resistance at higher speeds, while the narrower seat facilitates pedaling.
Expect to pay: $500 to more than $3,000. ————————

Features You have some choice in configuring a bike. See which variations you prefer.

Linear-pull brakes

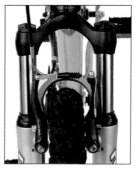

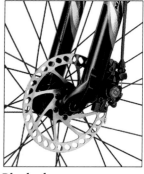

Disc brakes

Brakes

Long-arm cantilever brakes (V-brakes or linear-pull brakes) are fine for most uses. For rough, sloppy terrain, go with disc brakes, which will spare your wheel rims from the abrasion of muddy braking. Some bikes are sold with your choice of brakes. Discs add $100 or more. You can retrofit some bikes with discs; ask at the bike shop. Bikes with disc brakes: 10, 11, 12, 13, and 14. (11 and 12 can be bought with linear-pull brakes, for $100 less.)

Handlebars

High-rise handlebars let you sit fairly upright. With low-rise and flat handlebars, you lean forward. Road bikes use drop bars for an aerodynamic bent-over position. See which position feels best. Most handlebars can be raised or lowered, and adjustable-angle stems give more play. If you can't get comfortable, consider replacing the handlebars with a different type.

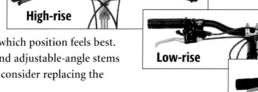

High-rise

Low-rise

Flat

Shifters

Twist shifters are collars on the handlebars that you twist to change gears. Trigger shifters have one lever for upshifting and one for downshifting, one pair each for the front and rear gears. Neither type is inherently better. Most are indexed, meaning they click as you shift, so you don't have to guess where the next gear is. Bikes with twist shifters: all the tested comfort bikes (18, 19, 20, 21, 22, 23, and 24).

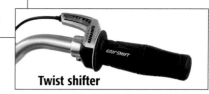

Trigger shifter

Twist shifter

Saddle

The narrow, firm seats on some mountain and road bikes let you change position and pedal more efficiently and provide more support. Comfort bikes and many hybrids have wider, softer seats, often with a suspension seatpost. If you don't like a seat, get one with a different shape, more or less padding, or channels or cutouts to ease pressure. Cost: $25 and up.

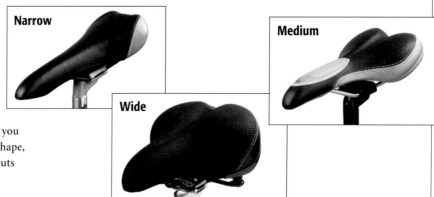

Narrow

Medium

Wide

Gearing

Most bikes have 3 front gears and 7 to 10 rear gears, yielding 21 to 30 speeds. Bikes priced at $1,000 and up will almost certainly have the appropriate number and range of gears. Don't expect decent gearing from cheap bikes. Where you need to compare models is in the midrange, where bike makers may compromise to keep the price low. The gearing on most midpriced models should be fine for flat or hilly pavement. To ease pedaling on steep dirt trails, look for 22 or fewer teeth on the small front gear and 32 or more on the large rear gear.

Features by model

Key no.	Model	Comes with disc brakes	Can add disc brakes	Adjustable fork suspension	Twist shifters	Suspension seatpost	Adjustable stem angle	Fork suspension lockout	Rear suspension lockout	Mount for rear luggage rack
1	**Cannondale** Jekyll 400		•	•					•	
2	**Specialized** FSR XC Pro		•	•				•		
3	**Trek** Fuel 80		•	•						
4	**Giant** NRS2		•	•						
5	**Gary Fisher** Sugar +4		•	•						
6	**Gary Fisher** Marlin		•	•						•
7	**Specialized** Rockhopper		•	•						•
8	**Trek** 4500		•	•						•
9	**Raleigh** M60		•	•						•
10	**Giant** Yukon	•		•						•
11	**Schwinn** Mesa GSD	•		•						•
12	**GT** Avalanche 2.0 Disc	•		•						•
13	**Mongoose** Rockadile ALD	•		•						•
14	**Giant** Cypress LX	•		•		•	•			•
15	**Jamis** Tangier			•		•				•
16	**Gary Fisher** Nirvana		•	•		•	•			•
17	**Specialized** Crossroads Elite			•		•	•			•
18	**Jamis** Explorer 2.0				•	•	•			
19	**GT** Timberline			•	•	•	•			
20	**Trek** Navigator 100				•	•				•
21	**Schwinn** Sierra GS				•	•				•
22	**Specialized** Expedition				•	•				•
23	**Raleigh** SC30				•	•				•
24	**Diamondback** Wildwood				•	•	•			•

Cheap bikes are not bargains

Wal-Mart and Toys "R" Us sell bikes from brands such as Huffy, Mongoose, Roadmaster, and Schwinn for $100 to $200. They seem like good deals, so why spend $300 or more?" Because you get what you pay for. Mass-market bikes have cheaper construction than higher-priced bikes and can weigh 7 or 8 pounds more. They come in only one size, so you're not likely to get a great fit. And mass merchants can't match bike shops for quality of assembly, expert advice, and service.

We tried out two full-suspension bikes and one front-suspension model from the big-box stores, priced at $120 to $230. Shifting of the full-suspension bikes' 21 speeds wasn't as smooth as on bike-shop models. Shock absorption and handling were fair to decent on pavement and on dirt paths, but these "mountain bikes" couldn't handle rough off-road terrain. On steep paved roads, the extra weight, poor gearing, and mushy suspensions made pedaling uphill very hard.

The front-suspension model did much better on pavement and on fairly smooth dirt trails—after we adjusted the setup.

Bike Ratings

Excellent = ◉ Very good = ◕ Good = ○ Fair = ◐ Poor = ●. Key numbers with a * indicate Quick Picks.

Within types, in preformnance order.

Key no.	Brand and model	Price	Overall score	Shifting	Braking (dry)	Braking (wet)	Handling	Shock absorption	Climbing	Number of men's sizes	Number of women's sizes	Weight (lb.)
	Full suspension mountain bikes: Best for serious off-road cycling. Scores for handling, shock absorption, and climbing are from off-road tests.											
1*	**Cannondale** Jekyll 400	$1,100	◉	◉	◕	◕	◉	◉	◉	4	–	32
2*	**Specialized** FSR XC Pro	1,200	◉	◕	◕	◉	◉	◉	◉	4	2	29.5
3*	**Trek** Fuel 80	1,150	◉	◉	◕	◕	◉	◕	◉	4	–	30
4*	**Giant** NRS 2	1,450	◕	◉	○	◕	◉	◕	◉	4	–	28.5
5	**Gary Fisher** Sugar +4	1,100	◕	◕	◕	◉	◕	◕	◉	4	–	31
	Front suspension mountain bikes: Best for moderate off-road cycling. Scores for handling, shock absorption, and climbing are from off-road tests.											
6*	**Gary Fisher** Marlin	$450	◕	◕	○	◉	◉	○	◉	5	–	29.5
7*	**Specialized** Rockhopper	440	◕	◕	◕	◉	◉	○	◉	6	3	29.5
8*	**Trek** 4500	440	◕	◕	◕	◉	◕	○	◉	7	3	30.5
9*	**Raleigh** M60	450	◕	○	○	◉	◕	○	◉	5	–	31.5
10	**Giant** Yukon	440	◕	◕	○	◉	○	◐	◉	6	–	31
11	**Schwinn** Mesa GSD	500	○	◕	◐	◕	◕	◐	◉	4	–	30.5
12	**GT** Avalanche 2.0 Disc	500	○	◕	◕	◕	◐	◕	5	–	31.5
13	**Mongoose** Rockadile ALD	400	○	◕	○	◕	○	●	◉	3	–	32
	Hybrid bikes: Best for moderate rides on pavement and smooth paths. Scores shown are from tests on pavement.											
14*	**Giant** Cypress LX	$470	◕	◕	○	◕	◕	◉	○	5	3	31.5
15*	**Jamis** Tangier	480	◕	◕	○	◕	○	◉	○	5	2	31
16*	**Gary Fisher** Nirvana	470	○	◕	○	◉	○	◕	○	5	3	31
17	**Specialized** Crossroads Elite	425	○	◕	◕	◉	◐	◕	○	4	2	31.5
	Comfort bikes: Best for casual neighborhood rides. Scores shown are from tests on pavement.											
18*	**Jamis** Explorer 2.0	$300	◕	◉	◕	◉	○	◉	◕	4	2	33
19*	**GT** Timberline	300	◕	◕	◕	◉	○	◕	◕	4	2	32.5
20*	**Trek** Navigator 100	300	◕	○	○	◕	○	◉	◕	4	3	35.5
21*	**Schwinn** Sierra GS	300	◕	◕	○	◉	○	◕	◕	4	2	32
22	**Specialized** Expedition	280	○	○	◕	◕	○	◕	◕	4	2	31.5
23	**Raleigh** SC30	290	○	◕	○	◕	○	◐	◕	5	2	33
24	**Diamondback** Wildwood	285	○	◐	○	○	◕	◉	◕	5	2	33.5

Chart originally appeared in the July 2004 issue of Consumer Reports.

GUIDE TO THE RATINGS **Brand and model:** All tested models have aluminum frame, suspension front fork, aluminum wheel rims, and riser handlebars. Most tested models have linear-pull brakes, medium-wide saddle, quick-release front and rear wheels and seatpost, and fittings for attaching two water bottles. **Overall score** is based on shifting, braking, handling, shock absorption, climbing, and weight. **Test results:** Shifting is ease and smoothness of changing gears. **Dry and wet braking** reflect stopping distance from a speed of 15 mph on dry and wet pavement. For mountain bikes, **handling** and **shock absorption** were tested on a rugged one-mile trail; **climbing** was tested on short, steep sandy and rocky trails. For comfort and hybrid bikes, **handling** was tested in moderate-speed turns on flat pavement and riding down a winding road at 25 mph; **shock absorption** was tested on moderately uneven road surfaces; and climbing was tested up a steep road. **Features:** Weight is to the nearest half-pound for an 18-inch men's frame or the closest size available to that. **Price** is approximate retail.

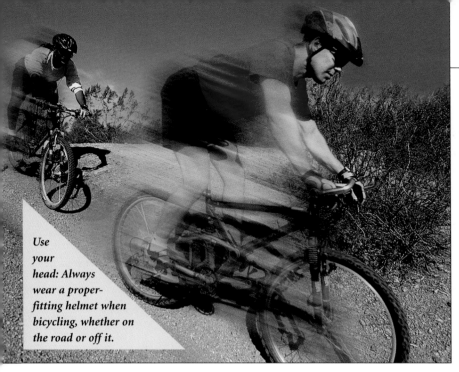

Use your head: Always wear a proper-fitting helmet when bicycling, whether on the road or off it.

Bike helmets: For safety's sake

Some bike helmets are getting better and easier to adjust, thanks to technological improvements appearing at all price levels. But several other helmets failed our tests because the buckle broke—a recurring problem we've noticed for years.

Designs have a safety edge. Most adult helmets in our tests, and others costing as little as $30, now use in-mold technology, in which impact-absorbing foam is bonded to the outer shell. After a crash, it's easy to see whether the helmet is dented and thus needs replacing. That's not always the case with helmets whose shell is taped or glued to the foam. The shell typically bounces back after a crash, so a damaged liner can be hard to see.

Helmets are easier to use. Most helmets now have easily adjustable straps to create a snug fit; many helmets for young riders also have buckles designed to avoid pinching the skin.

Beware of breaking buckles

Several models failed our tests. All bike helmets sold in the U.S. must meet federal safety standards for impact and buckle-and-strap system strength. Yet in our tests, buckles broke in multiple samples of two adult helmets and one toddler helmet. With the toddler helmet, 4 of 12 samples failed. With one adult helmet, 3 of 12 samples failed; with another, 2 of 12 failed. Our test applied a force slightly less than the federal standard.

The above models are called out in the "Ratings." We don't recommend buying them; if you already own one, consider replacing it with a highly rated helmet. Until you replace it, however, continue to wear it, since any helmet is better than nothing. The buckles at issue are the TSK-63 by ITW Nexus and the Ergo-Lok by National Molding. We can't pinpoint the cause of the problems; other helmets that use those same buckles passed our tests.

How to choose

Try it on before you buy. If you need help getting a good fit, consider buying your helmet at a bike shop, which may offer better service than other retailers.

Don't lose your cool. If you ride a lot, look for a helmet that did well in our ventilation tests. Many youth helmets aren't well ventilated, so an avid young cyclist might do better with a smaller-sized adult model.

Want a multisport helmet? "Skate style" helmets, which cover more of the head, look like they'd be appropriate for other sports, but many are not. Only helmets that meet skateboard and snowboard standards are best suited for those sports. Helmets that meet skateboarding standards must withstand multiple impacts. Of the three skate-style helmets we tested (Bell Scuffle, Mongoose BMX, and W Ripper2) only the W Ripper2 is a multisport, multiple-impact helmet.

Know when to discard it. With all but a multiple-impact model, replace your helmet if you crash and hit your head.

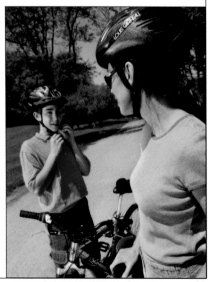

Kids are far likelier to wear a helmet when adults wear one, too, says a survey by the National Safe Kids Campaign and Bell Sports.

Helmet Ratings

Excellent = ◉   Very good = ◕   Good = ○   Fair = ◔   Poor = ●.   * indicate Quick Picks; † similar models.

Within types, in prerformnance order.

Key	Brand and model	Price	Overall	Impact	Retention	Ventilation	Ease of use
	Adult Helmets						
1* †	**Louis Garneau** Zen, Rev	$45	◕	◕	◉	◉	◉
2*	**Trek** Interval	60	◕	◕	◉	◕	◉
3	**Specialized** M1	60	◕	○	◉	◉	◕
4	**Giro** Pneumo	140	◕	○	◉	◉	◉
5	**Bell** X-Ray	100	◕	○	◉	◉	◉
6	**Bell** Ghisallo	100	◕	○	◉	◕	◉
7	**Bell** Aquilla	45	◕	○	◉	◕	◉
8†	**Giro** Torrent II, Atlas II, Venus II, Transit II, Kickfire II	40	◕	○	◉	○	◉
9†	**Bell** Ukon II, Bella II, Arc II,Cognito II, Craze II	35	◕	○	◉	◔	◉
10	**Serfas** Cosmos, Curva, Flea	35	○	○	◉	○	◔
11	**Giro** Semi MX	60	○	○	◉	◔	◔
12*	**W** Ripper2 BMX/Skate	80	○	○	◉	●	◔
13	**Bell** Scuffle Wicked, Mirra Special Edition, X Games Backlash	25	◔	◔	◔	●	◔
14	**Specialized** Telluride NOT RECOMMENDED	60	◔	◕	●	◉	◕
15	**Bell** Influx NOT RECOMMENDED	60	◔	○	●	◕	◉
	Youth Helmets						
16*	**Specialized** Air Wave Mega	$30	◕	◉	◉	◔	◕
17	**Louis Garneau** Grunge 2-V	45	◕	◕	◉	○	◉
18	**Bell** Amigo	30	◕	◕	◉	◔	◉
19*	**Schwinn** Thrasher	20	◕	◕	◉	◔	◉
20	**Specialized** Airforce Youth	40	◕	○	○	◕	◉
21	**Bell** Deuce	30	◕	○	◉	◔	●
22	**Serfas** Rookie	30	○	○	◉	◔	●
23	**Mongoose** BMX Hardshell MG119	45	○	○	◉	●	◔
	Toddler Helmets						
24*	**Bell** Boomerang	$30	◕	◕	◉	◔	◕
25	**Giro** Me2 Rodeo	30	○	○	◉	◔	◕
26	**Schwinn** Toddler Value Pack Child Value Pack	20	○	○	◉	◔	◔
27	**Specialized** Kid Cobra	30	○	○	◕	●	◕
28	**Fisher-Price** Toddler Bell Bellino	20	◔	◔	◉	◔	●
29	**Trek** Little Dipper NOT RECOMMENDED	40	◔	○	●	○	◔

Chart originally appeared in the July 2004 issue of CONSUMER REPORTS.

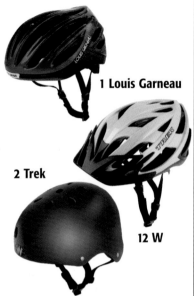

1 Louis Garneau

2 Trek

12 W

GUIDE TO THE RATINGS Brand and model: Many helmets can be replaced at a discount after being damaged in a crash. Louis Garneau, Serfas, and some Trek models can be replaced free of charge for one year; Specialized offers a voucher for a 20 percent discount for a new Specialized helmet. Bell charges $20 for some non-in-mold-shell models and $35 for some in-mold shell helmets. Fisher-Price, Giro, Mongoose, and Schwinn do not offer discounts. The **overall score** is based mainly on impact protection. **Test results: Impact** is how well each helmet absorbed energy in our impact test. **Retention** is how well the straps, buckles, and other hardware met our strength criteria. **Ventilation** is how well air flows through the helmet based on judgments by testers riding bicycles and our analysis of vent design. **Ease of use** is our judgment of how easily a helmet's straps, buckles, and other hardware could be adjusted. Price is approximate retail.

How to ensure the right fit

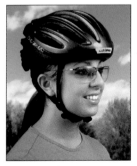
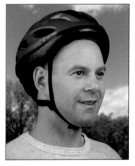

A bike helmet should sit level on your head (left), not tilted back like a hat (right).

Choosing a helmet that fits and wearing it properly increase your protection. Use the guidelines below:

• Use the appropriate foam pads and the rear stabilizer or helmet's fit system to create a snug (but not tight) fit when you place the helmet level on your head.

• With the chin strap buckled and all other straps tight, push up firmly on the helmet's front edge. If the helmet moves enough to expose the forehead, shorten the front straps, then tighten the chin strap enough so that you can feel the top of the helmet when you open your mouth. Repeat as necessary.

• Grasp the helmet by its rear edge and peel it off to the front. If it moves enough to cover your eyes, shorten the back straps (but leave the front straps alone). Repeat as necessary.

Bike racks: Tips for choosing the right one for you

The objective is simple. You want to carry your bicycle on your vehicle. But there's a seemingly dizzying selection of bike-rack styles and a wide range of prices from which to choose. In general, this is an advantage, but to get the right bike rack for your needs, you should do some research and compare the different makes and models. The right rack should fit the vehicle properly, securely transport the bikes, and fall within your budget. The wrong rack could be a safety hazard, scratch your vehicle, and possibly lead to a lost, stolen, or damaged bicycle.

CONSIDER YOUR NEEDS

The key to choosing the right bike rack is accurately defining your needs and assessing your current vehicles. Consider the following when choosing a bike rack:

- How often will you use it?
- How many bikes need to be transported?
- Will you need to change vehicles (e.g., switch the rack between husband's and wife's vehicles)?
- Is the vehicle leased or rented?
- How much are you willing to spend?
- How important is security?
- How high can you lift a bicycle by yourself, and hold it in position with one hand?
- Do you have a special bike, such as a tandem or one with an odd-shaped frame?
- Does your vehicle already have a tow hitch or roof-mounted utility rack? If so, what is the load capacity?

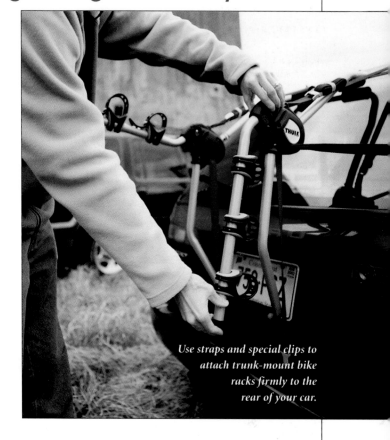

Use straps and special clips to attach trunk-mount bike racks firmly to the rear of your car.

- Does your vehicle have a rear-mounted spare tire that will interfere with certain types of mounts?
- Do you engage in other sports or activities, which may make one rack type more useful or cost-effective than another?

TYPES OF RACKS

Bike racks generally fall into three distinct categories: a strap-on trunk rack, a hitch-mount rack, and a roof rack. All types have good and bad points, but not all are available for every vehicle. The strap-on is the least expensive, but the least secure; the roof rack is the most versatile, but the most difficult to use; and the hitch-mount is the most expensive, but easy to operate. There are also specialty racks that are designed specifically for use with pickup trucks or for inside SUVs or vans. Some truck racks can be used above the bed, allowing for storage underneath. Others have specialty mounts that can be attached to rear-mounted spare tires and the rear ladders sometimes found on conversion vans.

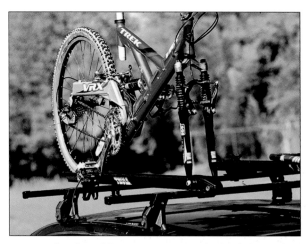

Some roof rack models require removing the bike's front wheel.

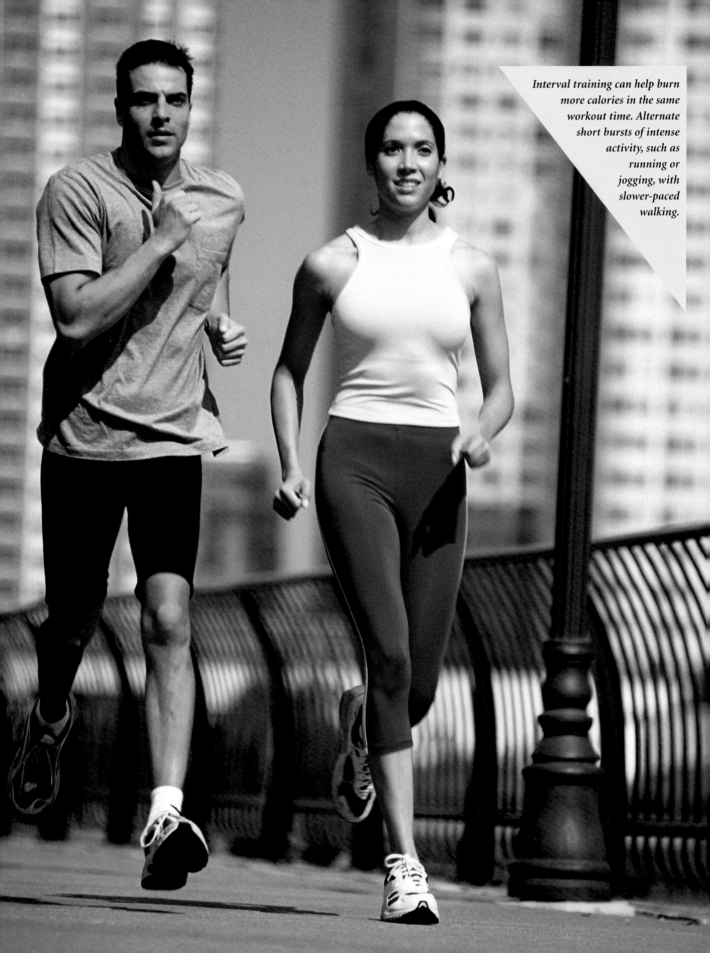

Interval training can help burn more calories in the same workout time. Alternate short bursts of intense activity, such as running or jogging, with slower-paced walking.

Make the most of your exercise minutes

P eople who want to get more from their workouts—or achieve the same benefits in less time—may think there's just one option: The brute-force approach of pushing your body harder, while enduring some monotonously repetitive exercise.

Fortunately, there are smarter, gentler, more interesting methods, two of them used by elite athletes, that can help even the least-fit individuals achieve their exercise goals by minimizing fatigue and boredom:

• Interval training, or bursts of vigorous exercise sandwiched between stretches of easier exercise that give your muscles a chance to recuperate.

• Cross-training, or switching off between different types of exercise, often within the same session.

• Finding creative, enjoyable ways to squeeze all sorts of physical activity into your daily routine.

This report will describe those efficient approaches to aerobic-style exercise, which can let you boost the speed, length, or frequency of your workouts without getting exhausted.

INTERVALS: MAKING HARD EASY

Vigorous workouts generally provide the most health benefits. But many people find them so hard or painful that they either quit or cut their sessions short before they can burn many calories or get much of the other benefits. Moderate exercise is usually more enjoyable, and most people can do it long enough to sig-nificantly improve certain important factors, such as blood pressure, blood sugar, and mood. But many individuals don't want to spend that much time working out. And some research suggests that even long moderate workouts won't significantly improve certain other fac-tors—such as aerobic fitness (the ability to do sustained,

Have a ball: Round out your workout routines by adding tennis, basketball, and other sports.

rapid activity), the "good" HDL cholesterol, and the risk of cancer—unless the pace is faster and harder than most people are used to.

Interval training combines the best of both approaches: The bursts of intense activity provide the advantages of vigorous exercise, while the moderate intervals give your muscles a break; that prevents lactic acid, a waste product of muscular activity, from reaching levels that make exercise painful and exhausting.

If you don't push yourself too hard, you're likely to exercise regularly.

"Someone who typically walks for, say, 30 minutes at a time will probably be able to do the same amount of interval training without feeling significantly more tired—but with far more benefits," says Richard Cotton, former chief exercise physiologist for the American Council on Exercise. For example, breaking up an exercise session so that you walk some of the time at a moderate 3.5-mph pace and an equal amount of time at a brisker 4.5-mph pace will burn roughly 30 percent more calories than walking moderately for the whole session. Similar benefits accrue when better-conditioned exercisers switch between, say, brisk walking and jogging. Those differences, multi-

plied over weeks and months, can translate into far more pounds lost as well as other health improvements.

Weaving surges of harder exercise into your workouts could also allow you to shorten your sessions and still achieve the same gains as before. Alternatively, that approach could let you do longer, more productive workouts. For example, suppose you can jog for about 30 minutes straight but feel exhausted afterward. If you alternated 5 minutes of jogging with 5 minutes of walking for a total of an hour, you'd still log 30 minutes of jogging, which yields the same cumulative benefits as the continuous run did. Moreover, you'd get the additional calorie burning and other benefits of the half hour of walking. Best of all, you'd probably feel less drained than after the shorter, unrelenting workout.

Interval training can help even poorly conditioned people, such as those whose disease limits their activities. For example, a recent study found that people with chronic obstructive pulmonary disease (either chronic bronchitis or emphysema) had to work out twice as long to achieve the same aerobic gains from traditional exercise classes as from interval training. Other research shows that such training is ideal for people with heart failure, since it challenges the muscles without straining the heart.

Caution: If you're recovering from major surgery or illness, have a chronic disease, or haven't exercised in years, check with your doctor before starting to work out, especially with intervals.

WHAT'S HARD?

For most people, the best way to determine the appropriate intensity of each interval is to assess the relative intensity, or "perceived exertion," of the exercise. Rate your

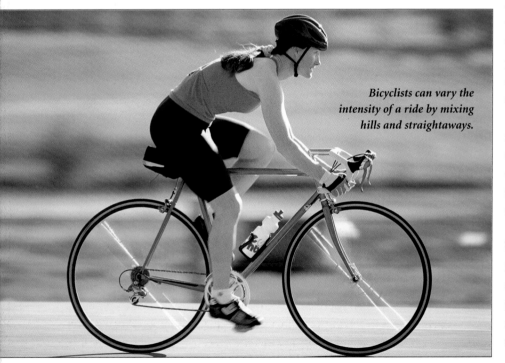

Bicyclists can vary the intensity of a ride by mixing hills and straightaways.

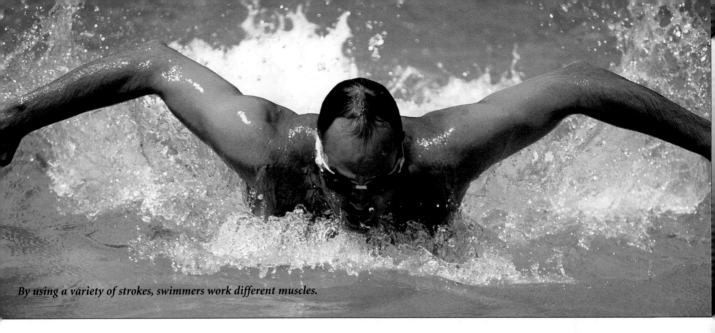

By using a variety of strokes, swimmers work different muscles.

exertion level on a scale of 6 (rest) to 20 (maximum effort, such as running all out for a bus). Beginners should generally alternate exercising between the light-to-fairly-hard range (9 to 11) and the somewhat hard (13 to 14) range. More experienced exercisers can bump up the intensity slightly, to 15 or so, and retreat to 11 or 12.

Of course, intensity is a relative term that only you can assess. A 12 is equivalent to the moderate effort required for, say, jogging by a young athlete or brisk walking by the average middle-aged person. For someone recovering from surgery or a long illness, interval training could mean alternating between simply moving at all and standing still. (Doctors may require people with certain underlying medical conditions to gauge their exercise intensity more precisely, by using a heart-rate monitor during the workout.)

You can also vary the intensity of your walks, runs, or rides by picking terrain that has a few hills; going downhill and on flat ground will give you a break after you've done the uphill work. Swimmers can alternate between demanding strokes, like the crawl, and more leisurely ones, such as the breast- or backstroke. (That approach, a cross-training technique, offers the added benefit of working slightly different muscles—see "Cross-training duos: good aerobic partners," on page 86.)

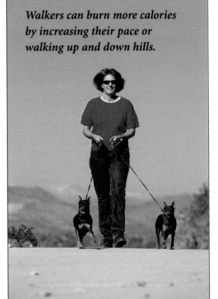

Walkers can burn more calories by increasing their pace or walking up and down hills.

The length of each interval doesn't really matter: Whether you do many short segments of vigorous activity or one or two long segments, it's the total of each type of exercise that counts.

You can determine the interval lengths by the distance traveled as well as the time spent. For example, you could push yourself hard from here to, say, the fifth telephone pole, tree, or parked car along your exercise route, then relax for the next five.

Whatever method you use to determine the intensity and length of the intervals, you're more likely to avoid problems and keep exercising regularly if you don't overextend yourself. "A common mistake is to turn interval training into a competition with yourself," Cotton says. "Don't let your ego take over and push you to exhaustion or pain. Start by doing less than you think you can, then slowly increase how long or hard you're working out until you get a sense of your limits."

CROSS-TRAINING: SHARE THE LOAD

While interval training mainly lets you work out harder, cross-training encourages longer and more frequent sessions by making exercise easier, safer, and more enjoyable.

Cross-training duos: good aerobic partners

This chart shows four different types of aerobic-style exercises that can be profitably paired as part of a well-rounded cross-training program: competitive sports, such as basketball, tennis, volleyball, and golf (without the cart); activities that mainly work the legs, such as walking, running, cycling, or skating; activities that mainly work the upper body, such as swimming and rowing; and gardening, a popular hobby that can offer a surprisingly good workout.

Each check indicates that the paired exercises have or can have complementary features—one demands continuous exertion, the other is intermittent, for example. (Boxes with no checks indicate that the two exercises share the same feature and thus are not complementary—for example, they're both high impact.) The table does not pair swimming or rowing with gardening because they're too similar in several key features to make a good cross-training match.

Note that you can profitably switch off within the leg-exercise group as well, from walking or running to skating or cycling. Walking or running works the calves and lower-front thigh muscles; skating works the inner and outer thigh muscles; and cycling works the front-thigh and hip muscles. Combining walking or running with cycling has one other advantage: The first two are weight-bearing exercises and thus particularly good for the bones, while cycling is much less so.

	Upper body/ lower body	Continuous/ not continuous	Low or no impact/ moderate or high impact	Weight bearing/ nonweight bearing	Solitary/ potentially social	Calming/ arousing	Mobile/ mainly stationary
Swimming or rowing + Activities that mainly work the legs	✔			✔	✔		
Swimming or rowing + Competitive sports	✔	✔	✔	✔	✔	✔	
Competitive sports + Activities that mainly work the legs		✔	✔		✔	✔	
Gardening + Activities that mainly work the legs	✔	✔		✔	✔		✔
Gardening + Competitive sports	✔		✔	✔	✔	✔	✔

Chart originally appeared in November 2003 issue of CONSUMER REPORTS on Health newsletter.

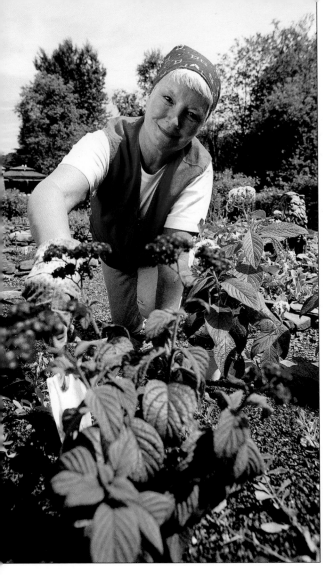

Active hobbies such as gardening can provide a boredom-beating alternative to just a single type of exercise.

Switching off among different activities within a single session—say, from a treadmill to a rowing machine to a stationary bike—minimizes weariness, since you don't work any muscles to exhaustion. Alternating exercises from day to day similarly cuts fatigue by giving the tired muscles a day off. Either approach—particularly if done with the interval method—allows you to lengthen your individual workouts, exercise more days of the week, or just enjoy easier sessions. Equally important, cross-training yields better overall fitness by working muscles throughout the body.

Moreover, cross-training lets you develop a diversified program that keeps boredom at bay, creates exercise options regardless of the season or weather, and reduces the risk of inflammation, strains, tears, and stress fractures caused by overusing a particular muscle, joint, or bone. Those advantages further encourage frequent, regular exercise.

It's particularly easy to cross-train at a health club, since you can hop from one exercise machine to another. But you can do it at home, too, without investing in machines. Consider not only the standard options such as walking, cycling, and swimming, but also sports (such as golf, softball, tennis, or volleyball) and active hobbies (such as dancing, gardening, and kite flying). Try to alternate among exercises that work different muscles or have complementary features, such as intermittent vs. continuous, fixed vs. mobile, gentle vs. jarring, calming vs. arousing, or solitary vs. social.

SQUEEZE IT IN

It's easier to get lots of exercise if you try to be physically active throughout the day. And every extra bit of physical activity helps, even if it's only a few minutes at a time. For example, studies have shown that disease and death rates go down as the total daily number of blocks walked or stairs climbed goes up.

Here are some ideas on how to squeeze physical activity into your day:

• Walk briskly at least part of the way to or from your workplace.

• Use stairs rather than escalators or elevators whenever possible.

• Take a brisk walk at lunchtime.

• Park at the far end of the parking lot when you go shopping.

• Bicycle to do errands or visit friends.

• Play actively—a game of tag, one-on-one basketball, a bike ride—with your children or grandchildren.

• Walk the dog. If you don't have a dog, borrow one.

• Ride a stationary bicycle while reading the newspaper.

• Work out on an exercise ball while watching television.

• Keep hand squeezers, dumbbells, elastic bands, or ankle weights near your desk at the office or at home. Exercise your hands, arms, or legs during breaks or while reading.

Treadmills: more for the money

Bad weather and barking dogs aren't the only reasons to consider joining the roughly 11 million Americans who do at least some of their walking or running indoors on a treadmill.

These motorized machines help you burn more calories than exercise bikes and are easier to use than stair climbers and ski machines. And because exercising on a treadmill is weight-bearing, it can help prevent the bone-weakening effects of osteoporosis.

Several new models provide more performance and features at about the same price as last year's. While you can still pay $3,000 or more, you'll find well-equipped machines for hundreds and even thousands of dollars less (see the "Ratings" chart on page 89).

Many of the features you'll see are designed to make workouts safer and less boring—a frequent complaint about treadmills. The major developments:

More variety. Even moderately priced models include electronic programs that vary your exercise routine by automatically adjusting the belt speed and incline to simulate hills, flats, sprints, and recovery jogs. Some

let you add your own programs and will adjust the speed, incline, or both based on feedback from a heart-rate monitor—another feature found on nearly all but the most basic models.

Market leader Icon Health and Fitness (maker of Image, NordicTrack, ProForm, Reebok, and Weslo models) lets you connect the treadmill to the Internet for free automated exercise programs. You can connect with a personal trainer, but at $30 or so per 45-minute session, it isn't cheap.

More coddling. Bottle holders for water and sport drinks are becoming as common on treadmills as cup holders in cars. Some models from NordicTrack and Reebok have cooling fans in the console. Most treadmills now have a reading shelf or a cubbyhole for a TV remote.

Friendlier designs. Kicking the motor housing and tripping used to be a common risk, especially for users with a long stride, since the housing was higher than the belt's forward edge.

Most treadmills now have a hous-

The $2,800 LifeFitness T3i was one of the highest-rated treadmills in our survey.

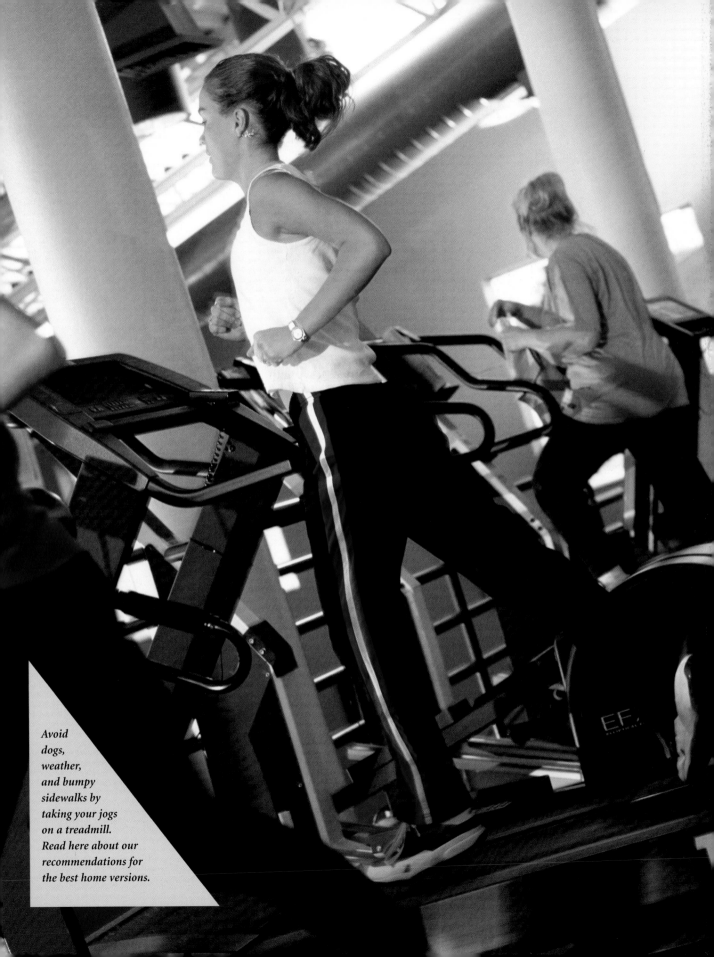

Avoid dogs, weather, and bumpy sidewalks by taking your jogs on a treadmill. Read here about our recommendations for the best home versions.

Choose a price range based on your exercise needs

Treadmills fall into three broad price groups based on how well they're built and the number of features they include. Consider the exercise you or family members do most. Then use the information below to decide how much treadmill you need.

Basic: $300 to $700
Best for walkers on a budget.

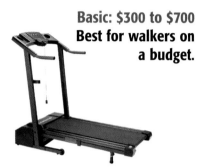

Typically include a 10-mph top speed; a 10 percent maximum incline; displays of speed, distance, time, and calories; a shelf and water-bottle holders; and folding deck. But these often aren't large or sturdy enough for running, and the deck may not decline flat—a problem for less-fit users.

Midrange: $800 to $1,800
Best for walkers and occasional runners.

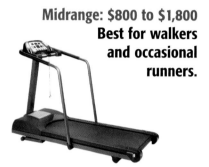

Typically include the same features as basic treadmills, plus a heart-rate monitor, exercise programs, and a deck that declines completely flat. But some don't fold. And durability may be an issue if you share it with serious runners.

High end: $2,000 to $3,500
Best for frequent, dedicated runners.

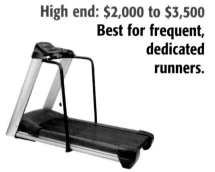

Typically include the same as midrange machines, plus the sturdier deck and frame, and the more powerful motor required for frequent fast running. But most high-end models are large and lack a folding deck, a potential problem if the exercise room for your treadmill is small.

---

ing that's relatively flush with the belt or use a concave housing, with a console and handrails mounted farther back to prevent kicking the housing.

HOW TO CHOOSE

Effective workouts without a steep learning curve help explain why treadmills are less likely than other fitness machines to become clothes racks. Different treadmills serve different needs, however. We found that some are built for the added pounding of running, while others are better for gentler walks.

Start by deciding whether you want a treadmill for walking, running, or both (see "Choose a price range based on your exercise needs," above), since a higher price and added sturdiness tend to go hand in hand. Then consider these points before buying:

Put programs into perspective. You may want lots of them if you run regularly or need varied routines to hold your interest. If not, you may be able to save money on a simpler model. Also consider skipping pricier machines that offer a 15-percent incline or 12-mph top speed if you prefer less-strenuous workouts.

Look for safety. Features include critical components that make some treadmills safer than others. Look for foot rails wide enough for you to stand on comfortably when getting on and off. Be sure that the belt is long and wide enough for your speed and stride. Also check that the machine can hold your weight; some limit users to 250 pounds.

Be wary of horsepower claims. A lower-stressed, higher-horsepower belt motor is likely to perform better and last longer. Some treadmill manufacturers imply more power than they deliver by listing peak horsepower, rather than the continuous-duty power we list in our Ratings. Look for at least 2 continuous-duty hp for running.

Consider an extended warranty. The price and hassle of repairs make this often-frivolous coverage worth it, especially for models warranted for less than a year. See that in-house service is included.

Treadmill Ratings

Excellent = ◉   Very good = ◕   Good = ○   Fair = ◒   Poor = ●.

Similar models in smaller type, comparable to tested model. Most models at stores through January 2005. In performance order.

Key	Brand & model	Price	Belt (L x W, in.)	Motor hp	Overall score	Controls	Exercise flexibility	Ergonomics	Construction	Chest-strap heart monitor	Folding deck
							Test results			Features	
1	**Landice** Pro Sports Trainer L7	$2,900	58x20	3.0	◕	◕	◕	◕	◕		
2	**True** 400HRC	2,200	54x20	2.75	◕	◕	◕	◕	◕	✔	
3	**Life Fitness** T3i T3	2,800	52x20	2.3	◕	◕	◕	◕	◕	✔	
4	**Precor** M 9.33	3,500	58x20	2.75	◕	○	◕	◕	◕	✔	
5	**Life Fitness Sport** ST55 Essential FT6	1,800	52x20	2.0	◕	◕	◕	◕	◕	✔	✔
6	**Schwinn** 820p CR Best Buy	1,300	51x20	2.0	◕	◕	◕	◕	◕	✔	
7	**StarTrac** TR901	3,200	50x19	2.0	◕	◕	◕	◕	◕	✔	
8	**Nautilus** NTR 500††	2,300	56x20	2.7	◕	◕	◕	○	◕	✔	
9	**Vision Fitness** T9200 CR Best Buy	1,350	52x20	2.0	◕	◕	◕	◕	◕		
10	**Reebok** RX 9200†††	2,000	59x19	3.0	◕	◕	◕	◕	◕	✔	✔
11	**EVO by Smooth Fitness** EVO2	2,600	60x20	3.0	◕	◕	○	◕	○	✔	
12	**Image** 10.0†	400	50x18	1.3	◕	◕	○	○	◒		✔
13	**Weslo** Cadence 450†	300	47x16	1.3	○	◕	○	○	◒		✔
14	**Weslo** Cadence 70e†	280	47x16	1.3	○	○	◒	◒	◒		✔

† Weight limit is 250 lbs. †† Can be turned on without safety key, a concern with kids. ††† Discontinued, but still available.

GUIDE TO THE RATINGS Brand & model: All tested models have a safety key. Wheels for transport. Most tested models: Have a deck that lies flat at lowest incline. Weight limit above 250 pounds. Warranty of at least 1 year on labor, 2 years on parts. **Overall score** is based mainly on controls, exercise flexibility, ergonomics, and construction, including durability, using an accelerated-use test. **Belt** is the usable exercise surface; bigger is better. **Motor hp** denotes continuous horsepower, rather than peak, as supplied by the manufacturer. **Controls** reflects how easily users can adjust incline and belt speed, read the display, and select programs. **Exercise flexibility** denotes the range of incline and speed, stability, how flat the deck lies, and heart-rate-monitor effectiveness. **Ergonomics** factors include design of the belt area, foot rails, handrails, motor housing, safety features, and folding mechanism. **Construction** denotes mostly motor horsepower, wiring, hardware and weld quality, deck thickness, and durability. **Price** is approximate retail. (Chart originally appeared in the Feb. 2004 issue of CONSUMER REPORTS.)

Treadmills and kids: a risky mix

More than 25,000 children in the United States are injured on treadmills and other exercise equipment each year, according to statistics compiled by the Consumer Product Safety Commission. In a study at The Children's Hospital of Philadelphia, abrasions were the most common injury, when hands were caught in the machine where the belt wraps around the rear roller. Half of those injuries occurred while an adult used the treadmill.

Adults are also at risk. Michael Bennett, a Minnesota Vikings running back, missed part of the 2003 National Football League season because of a treadmill injury. Overexertion can raise heart-attack and other risks, especially for those age 40 and up.

To safeguard yourself and your family:

- Keep children and pets away.
- Tether the safety key to your clothing when using a treadmill, then keep it out of a child's reach when you're done with your workout.
- Begin by standing on the treadmill's side rails. Then be sure that the belt is moving at a slow, safe speed before you step onto it.
- Check with a doctor before using a treadmill or any other exercise equipment regularly, particularly if you're over 40 or have health problems.
- Don't overdo it. If you can't talk without gasping for air, you're working too hard.

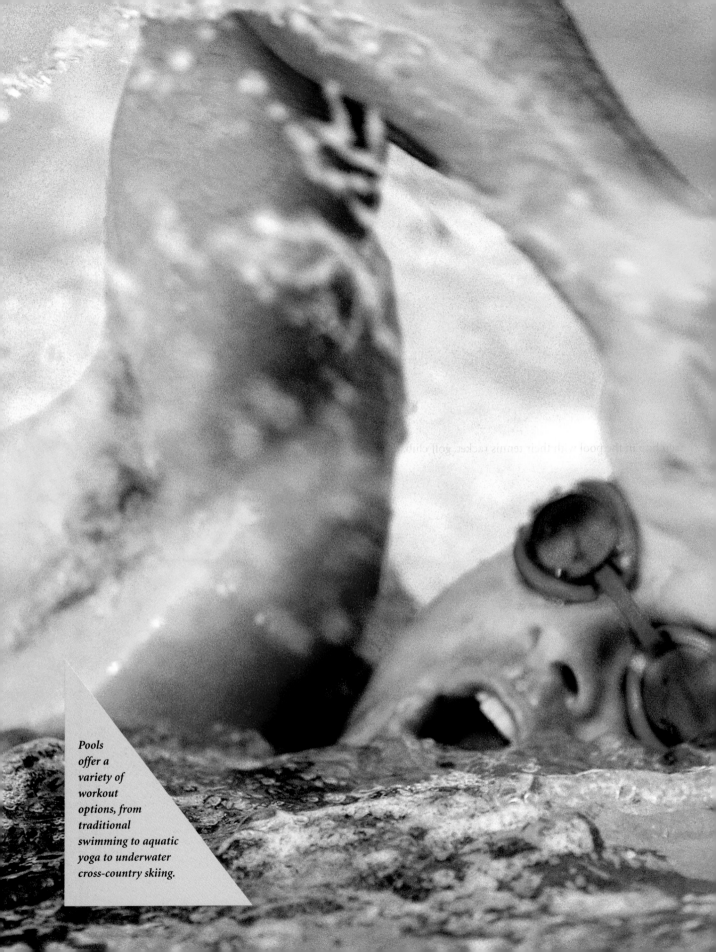

Pools offer a variety of workout options, from traditional swimming to aquatic yoga to underwater cross-country skiing.

Everyone
in the
pool

Until recently, the idea of exercising in water may have conjured up unappealing images: at best, swimming endless laps; at worst, undergoing physical therapy for an injury, disease, or disability. But today, swimming pools are overflowing with healthy people performing everything from aquatic yoga, kick boxing, and tae kwon do, to bicycling and cross-country skiing on submerged machines. Some people even hop in the pool with their tennis racket, golf club, or baseball bat, to strengthen and hone their swings.

"Certain water exercises may be passing fads," says Jane Katz, Ed.D., a professor of physical education and athletics at the City University of New York and a water-fitness pioneer. "But aquatic workouts, in one form or another, are here to stay. There are just so many benefits."

In a 2002 study Japanese researchers found that volunteers ages 60 to 75 who performed basic water workouts three times a week for 12 weeks improved in all three major measures of physical fitness: aerobic capacity, flexibility, and strength; they also reduced their body fat and cholesterol levels.

Other research suggests that walking, running, or doing aerobics in water can provide a generally more effective workout than the same exercises on land. It's also safer—a particular advantage for overweight, pregnant, or frail individuals and those with back or joint problems. Equally important, just being in a pool is cooling, energizing, and, because of the buoyancy, literally uplifting. So aquatic exercises seem less tedious and draining than their gravity-bound counterparts. Running in a pool, for example, can feel a little like bounding in slow motion across the surface of the moon.

In "The water workout" (page 97), we explain how to walk or jog effectively in water, and we describe four water calisthenics that you can do on your own. In the main report, we lay out the multiple benefits of water workouts and tell how to get your feet wet in an aquatics program.

WATER FEATURES

Aquatic exercises essentially use water as a piece of exercise equipment. "The greater resistance of water compared to air, combined with its buoyancy, offers benefits that are often harder and sometimes almost impossible to get on land," says John Spannuth, president of the United States Water Fitness Association. Specifically, exercising in water:

• **Protects the joints.** As you walk on land, your foot strikes the ground with the force of two to five times your weight. That impact can strain your back, hips, knees, and ankles. Standing still, you weigh twice as much on land as in waist-deep water, 10 times as much as in shoulder-deep water.

• **Combines aerobics with strength training.** Aquatic walking, jogging, or aerobics boost not only cardiovascular capacity but also strength, as you force your arms and legs

Aquatic jogging builds cardiovascular endurance and strength.

through the water, which offers roughly 10 times more resistance to motion than air does.

• **Builds multiple muscles.** Since water provides resistance in all directions, more muscles get exercised. For example, straight-leg lifts on land tone only the quadriceps, the front thigh muscle. But leg lifts in the water also strengthen the hamstrings, on the back of the thigh, as you press your leg down.

• **Offers a fast, vigorous workout.** Since you have to work harder to move through water, you can get a better aerobic workout than from similar "dry" exercises done in an equal amount of time—or get comparable benefits from a shorter workout. And the cooling, stimulating effect of the water, plus the reduced strain on the joints, encourages you to work out harder than you normally would.

Note that your heart rate in the water will be lower than usual, since the water pressure and other factors reduce the heart's pumping speed. So if you use heart rate to measure exercise intensity, lower your target rate by about 10 beats per minute. Or gauge intensity by your perceived exertion; safe and effective exercise should feel somewhat hard but not make breathing or talking difficult.

• **Promotes weight loss.** Since you can work out harder in water, you can burn more calories. And because water workouts are more comfortable, you're likely to exercise longer, increasing your total caloric expenditure.

However, swimming may not be as good as other water exercises for weight loss. Most novices cannot swim long enough to burn many calories. And overweight people have to work extra hard to get a good workout while swimming, since their excess body fat lets them float more easily.

• **Improves flexibility.** You can often assume positions in the water that can be difficult to reach on land; that can help you boost your flexibility, especially if you have stiff or painful joints. For example, people with arthritic hips may find they are able to lift their legs higher because of the buoyancy of water, allowing them to expand their hips' range of motion.

• **Lets you move with control and precision.** It's easier to move slowly in water; that allows you to perfect your technique in certain sports or martial arts.

One important caution: Don't substitute water workouts for all of the exercises you do on land: Weight-bearing exercises help prevent bone loss better than water exercises can.

WHAT YOU NEED

Cotton sneakers (with nonmarking soles) provide good traction and extra support in and around the pool. But drying them can be inconvenient. Water shoes—which give comparable traction and often cost less than sneakers and dry much faster—are usually preferable.

Special webbed gloves, paddles, fins, and other paraphernalia can add variety to your workouts and boost their intensity. But before you invest in equipment, try using only what nature provided you.

If you're prone to swimmer's ear, an ear-canal infection caused by trapped water, try using ear plugs. If water does get trapped, use this technique: Tip your head to the side, with the wet ear upward, pull the ear up and back, and empty a dropper of rubbing alcohol into the canal. (That helps evaporate the water.) Wiggle or pull your ear to coax the drops all the way in, then tip your head to the other side to let the ear drain. (Don't do this if you have a ruptured eardrum or a tympanostomy tube.)

The water workout

Signing up for a class is a good way to ease into water exercise. Health clubs and local chapters of the Y or the Arthritis Foundation frequently offer such classes. (To find those chapters, look in the phone book or online at *www.ymca.net* or *www.arthritis.org.*) Here, we tell how to get started on your own. Beginners should start with 15- to 20-minute sessions and slowly increase their length and intensity.

WATER WALKING

Walking or jogging in the pool can exercise both your upper and lower body.

- Start in waist-deep water; work up to deeper water as you get in better shape.
- Fight the tendency to stay on your tiptoes in the water, since that stresses the lower legs; instead, put your heel down first.
- Don't lean forward.
- Swing your arms, and keep them closer to your body than you would on land.
- To work your muscles evenly, walk or jog forward and backward for equal amounts of time. You can also work muscles more fully by moving sideways.

WATER AEROBICS

The following exercises, recommended by Jane Katz, Ed.D. work the muscles in the upper body, midsection, and legs. You can do them alone, or mix in some walking and jogging to add variety and intensity.

Leg swings. Stand with your back against the corner of the pool, one hand on either edge. Lift your legs to create an "L" with your body. Then swing your legs from side to side. If that's too hard, try it with your knees bent.

Leg lifts. Stand in water that's slightly above your waist, with your back against the wall of the swimming pool. Lift your legs one at a time as high as they'll comfortably go, keeping your legs straight. For an easier workout, bend the knee of the leg you're lifting before each lift. To increase the resistance, use a special float (a "pull buoy") attached to your ankle.

Arm swirls. Stand in shoulder-deep water, then bend your knees slightly so that your arms and shoulders are fully submerged. Extend your arms out to the side and rotate them forward in a circular motion, then backward. You can increase the intensity by flexing your wrists up and down; by cupping your hands to increase resistance; by making larger, more vigorous circles; or by walking or jogging as you move your arms.

Jumping jacks. Stand in chest-deep water with your arms at your sides and your feet together. Rotate your palms forward. Keeping your arms straight, force them up out of the water and touch your palms overhead. At the same time, jump up to spread your legs in an inverted "V" position. Then turn your palms outward and bring your arms back to your sides as you bring your legs back together.

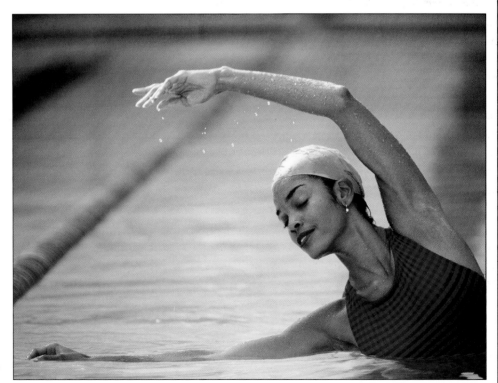

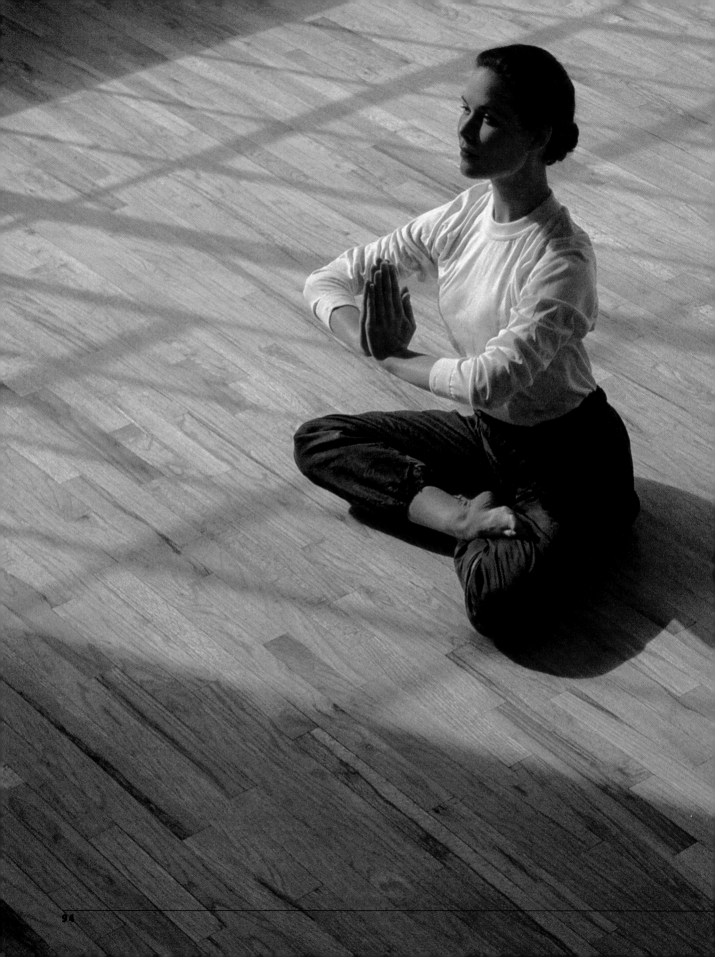

Health & Wellness

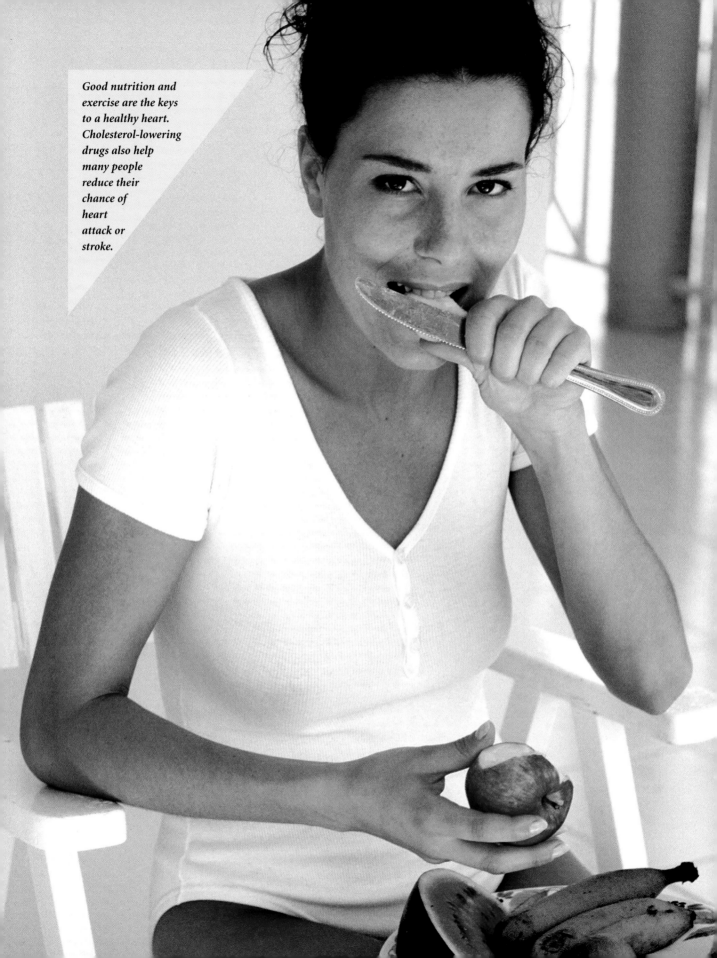

Good nutrition and exercise are the keys to a healthy heart. Cholesterol-lowering drugs also help many people reduce their chance of heart attack or stroke.

Cholesterol: how low should you go?

In 2001 public-health experts set aggressive new cholesterol guidelines that nearly tripled the number of people who should be taking cholesterol-cutting drugs to almost one-fifth of all adults. Now many experts suspect that even those goals probably aren't aggressive enough.

One reason: People at high coronary risk who reduced their "bad" LDL cholesterol to well below the 2001 target level stopped artery clogging from getting worse in one study and slashed their risk of heart attack and stroke in another. Moreover, research suggests that certain relatively new risk factors may increase many people's cardiovascular risk to the point where they, too, should consider sharply cutting their cholesterol levels.

That evidence suggests that many more people may need to take cholesterol-lowering drugs and that many of those already on them may need to boost the dosages, switch to a stronger drug, or try multiple medicines.

But that call for more-aggressive treatment comes when few people are meeting even the 2001 cholesterol goals. While new drugs could make reaching lower levels easier, their long-term safety remains unknown. And the uncertainty extends beyond drugs: A flurry of research, best sellers, and other publicity has convinced many Americans that the low-fat diet recommended for reducing cholesterol levels, with or without medication, may not be best after all.

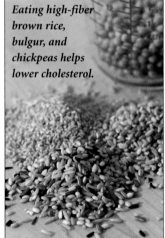

Eating high-fiber brown rice, bulgur, and chickpeas helps lower cholesterol.

THE LOWER THE BETTER?

Cholesterol travels through the bloodstream as part of larger particles known as lipoproteins. Treatment for elevated cholesterol levels focuses on low-density lipoprotein (LDL), which tends to dump its cholesterol load into the artery walls. Whether and how much you need to lower your LDL level depends in part on your overall coronary risk, which is determined by your LDL plus other established risk factors such as diabetes, high blood pressure, smoking, and a family history of heart disease, according to the 2001 guidelines. (To determine your risk and to read the guidelines, go to *www.nhlbi.nih.gov/guidelines/cholesterol/index.htm.*)

The research, while preliminary, suggests that starting cholesterol medication at less-elevated LDL levels and aiming lower than those guidelines mandate may often be worthwhile, especially for people at highest risk. A large British clinical study published in 2002 found that giving medication to high-risk people reduced their chance of heart attack or stroke by roughly 25 percent. Risk fell

Do home cholesterol tests work?

Comprehensive cholesterol screening should be a regular part of your medical checkups. But should you also test cholesterol at home with a kit available from the pharmacy or via the Internet?

Our advice, after testing five widely sold kits: Don't bother.

Two were inaccurate. Three test only for total cholesterol and so provide less information than most people need. All require you to draw a relatively large amount of blood. And none save you much money.

We compared the five kits with results from a hospital lab, using blood from staff volunteers. Here's what we found:

• The CholesTrak, First Check, and Home Access kits (the same kit from three companies) were judged good; all readings varied no more than 15 percent from those at the hospital. However, those three kits measure only total cholesterol, which isn't necessarily the most meaningful indicator. A full lipid profile, also measuring HDL ("good") cholesterol and triglycerides, is far more informative. A full profile yields the most important figure, LDL ("bad") cholesterol levels.

• The CardioChek (which costs $185) and the Biosafe Cholesterol Panel mail-in kit deliver a full lipid profile. But both yielded results that were often wide of the mark.

• The CardioChek requires you to draw blood three times from your fingers for a complete lipid profile. With the others, you need only one finger prick. But they all require 45 to 100 microliters of blood. Drawing the necessary blood can be difficult, painful, and messy. By contrast, a blood-glucose test needs only 1 to 3 microliters.

• The cost of an at-home test ranges from $14 for the First Check to about $30 for the Biosafe Cholesterol Panel. A full profile at the doctor's office and any needed follow-up tests will cost about $30 each. They're usually covered by health insurance. The home kits aren't covered.

Leaving much to be desired: Kits like the CholesTrak don't provide enough information. The CardioChek and the Biosafe were inaccurate.

significantly even in those who had an initial LDL level below 100 milligrams per deciliter (mg/dl)—the guidelines' threshold for starting drug treatment in high-risk people—and who then got their LDL down to an average of 65 mg/dl. Another clinical trial, presented at the American Heart Association's annual meeting in 2003, found that arterial plaque deposits stopped expanding only in an aggressively treated group that got its average LDL level down to 79 mg/dl.

Our medical consultants say that people at high coronary risk who have an LDL level above 100 mg/dl should

People at high coronary risk should limit cholesterol-rich eggs and fatty meats.

almost certainly start drug therapy in addition to making lifestyle changes. Those individuals—as well as others at similar risk whose LDL is already below 100 mg/dl—should talk with their doctor about whether to aim for a lower level.

A more aggressive approach may also be justified in people who are at moderate coronary risk based on standard risk factors but have other, less established factors, too. Those include elevated C-reactive protein (CRP), a marker of arterial inflammation; elevated homocysteine, an artery-damaging amino acid; and arterial calcium deposits (seen on a CT scan), which correlate fairly well with plaque buildup. Experts believe elevations in any of those factors may vault otherwise moderate-risk individuals into a higher-risk group and thus justify aggressive cholesterol-cutting therapy. Again, that's a decision each person must make with his or her doctor.

Our experts say people at high coronary risk with a "bad" LDL cholesterol level above 100 mg/dl should almost certainly start drug therapy.

ally quite safe, their risks rise at higher doses. And little is known about the long-term safety of the newer drugs, specifically ezetimibe (Zetia) and rosuvastatin (Crestor).

So people taking such drugs need to know the potential adverse effects and contact their doctor at the first sign of any problem. Moreover, taking the maximum recommended dose may be unwise. Studies show that the highest doses often provide minimal additional benefits while substantially increasing the chance of adverse effects.

TREAT AGGRESSIVELY–BUT SAFELY

To reach LDL levels below 100 mg/dl, patients will likely have to take cholesterol-lowering medications known as "statins," either alone or in combination with other drugs that can also reduce LDL levels, as well as improve other risk factors for heart disease such as a low level of the "good" HDL cholesterol. While cholesterol drugs are gener-

Instead, it often makes sense to add a second medication. For example, doubling the dose of a "statin" drug, such as atorvastatin (Lipitor) or lovastatin (Mevacor), on average lowers LDL cholesterol only an additional 6 percent. But adding a complementary medication, such as

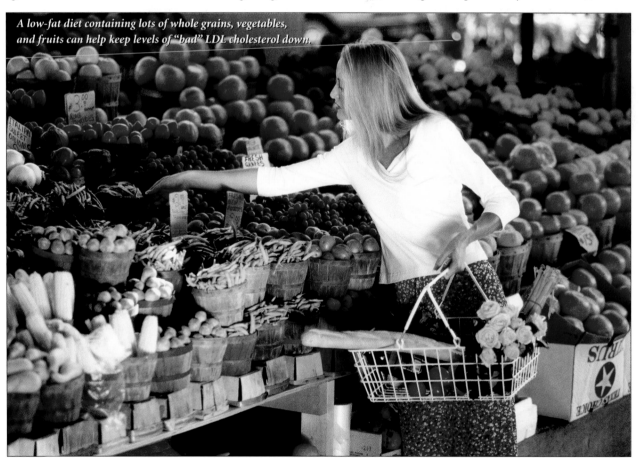

A low-fat diet containing lots of whole grains, vegetables, and fruits can help keep levels of "bad" LDL cholesterol down.

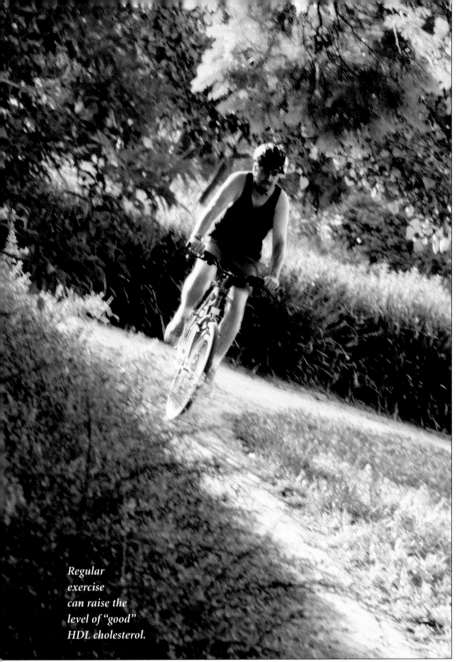

Regular exercise can raise the level of "good" HDL cholesterol.

unsaturated fat, found mainly in nontropical vegetable oils, may help control weight and improve cholesterol and triglyceride levels; eating lots of refined grains may have the opposite effects.

But the traditional cholesterol-lowering diet and other steps still play a central role in protecting the heart. Indeed, despite the new emphasis on medication, some people with a high LDL can still get by with lifestyle steps alone. And all people who take the drugs must make those changes too, since they're unlikely to reach their goals otherwise and because those steps protect the heart in many other ways as well.

Specifically, they should adopt the healthy habits listed below. (Consult food labels or the U.S. Department of Agriculture's food-composition Web page, *www.nal.usda.gov/fnic/foodcomp*, to track your intake of each of the following food components.)

• Reduce intake of saturated fat, found mainly in animal foods, to less than 7 percent of total calories. (To learn how much saturated fat that means for you, go to the National Cholesterol Education Project's diet-information Web page at *www.nhlbisupport.com/chd1/create.htm*.) And minimize your intake of trans fat, found in foods containing partially hydrogenated oil, such as most margarines and many fast or packaged foods. However, you don't have to consume less unsaturated fat unless you have difficulty limiting your total caloric intake.

• Consume less than 200 milligrams per day of cholesterol, the amount in about one egg yolk, 10 ounces of lean sirloin, or 8 ounces of skinless chicken breast.

• Consume lots of fiber, mainly from whole grains, fruits, vegetables, and beans. Women should aim for 25 grams a day up to age 50, and 21 grams after that age; men in those age groups should aim for 38 and 30 grams respectively.

• Lose excess weight by cutting calories and exercising.

ezetimibe, can cut it by 17 to 24 percent. A second drug may be appropriate when you have not only a high level of the "bad" LDL cholesterol but also either a low level of the "good," high-density lipoprotein (HDL) cholesterol (which drags cholesterol out of the arteries) or a high level of triglycerides, fats in the blood that elevate coronary risk.

LIFESTYLE CHANGES: STILL VITAL

Many Americans, infatuated with high-fat, low-carbohydrate diets, have concluded that the standard lifestyle advice for heart health doesn't work. It's true that the message has changed somewhat: Modest amounts of

A guide to cholesterol-lowering drugs

Statin drugs reduce levels of the "bad" LDL cholesterol more than other medications do, so they're the first choice for most people with elevated LDL. Statins may also help prevent heart attack and stroke by stabilizing plaque deposits and improving blood flow. (In addition, some evidence suggests that they may reduce the risk of Alzheimer's and kidney diseases, cancer, macular degeneration, and osteoporosis.) Other cholesterol drugs should be used when statins alone are insufficient or contraindicated, or possibly when levels of triglycerides or the "good" HDL cholesterol are abnormal.

Drug	Monthly cost*	Consider using when...	Precautions
STATINS			
Atorvastatin (*Lipitor*) **Fluvastatin** (*Lescol*) **Lovastatin** (generic, *Altoprev, Mevacor*) **Pravastatin** (*Pravachol*) **Simvastatin** (*Zocor*)	$51-$262	LDL level is elevated. Generic lovastatin is often preferred when LDL must be cut by less than 50 percent since it's cheaper and just as effective as others for moderate reductions and has a longer safety record. Atorvastatin is often preferred for those who need more than a 50 percent drop, since it's more powerful than others.	• Undergo liver-enzyme tests soon after therapy starts and possibly periodically thereafter. • Watch for muscle aches, which may indicate serious problems. • Don't take with cyclosporine or certain antibiotics and antifungals. • Use with particular caution when taking fenofibrate or gemfibrozil (see below).
Rosuvastatin (*Crestor*)	$76	Other statins (which have longer safety records) don't lower LDL enough.	• Rosuvastatin not recommended for Asians, who may face higher risk from the drug.
OTHER DRUGS			
Ezetimibe (*Zetia*)	$68	Statins are inappropriate or insufficiently effective alone.	Avoid if you have liver problems.
Bile-acid resins **Cholestyramine** (generic, *Questran*) **Colesevelam** (*Welchol*) **Colestipol** (*Colestid*)	$51-$157	Same as above. (Colesevelam is better tolerated and more convenient than other resins, but more expensive.)	• Increased fiber intake may relieve constipation and bloating, two common side effects. • Cholestyramine and colestipol can impair absorption of other drugs, so take them 1-2 hours after those drugs.
Niacin (generic, *Niacor, Niaspan*)	$9-$51	HDL level is low and possibly when triglyceride level is high; add to statin when LDL is also high.	To reduce flushing and other side effects, start with a low dose and consider taking aspirin 30 to 60 minute before niacin.
Fibrates **Fenofibrate** (*Lofibra, Tricor*) **Gemfibrozil** (generic, *Lopid*)	$50-91	Triglyceride level is high and possibly when HDL is low. Add to statin when LDL is also high. (Gemfibrozil doesn't lower triglycerides as much and is riskier, especially with a statin.)	Use with particular caution when taking a statin or antidiabetic or anticoagulant drugs, since fibrate can increase their effects.

*Cost data from "Rosuvastatin—A New Lipid-Lowering Drug," the Medical Letter on Drugs and Therapeutics, Oct. 13, 2003; and "Drugs for Lipid Disorders," Treatment Guidelines from the Medical Letter, August 2003. Price ranges reflect differences between initial and maximum dosages, brands, or generic and brand-name drugs. Costs rounded to nearest whole dollar. Chart originally appeared in the March 2004 issue of CONSUMER REPORTS on Health newsletter.

Consuming lots of fiber and moderate amounts of unsaturated fat may help by curbing hunger.

• Regardless of your weight, work out regularly. Exercise can raise the HDL level and may help lower LDL as well.

• Consider consuming about 2 grams a day of plant sterols or sterol derivatives, from products such as Benecol and Take Control margarine, and about 25 grams of soy protein from soy foods (though the evidence is weaker for soy than for sterols).

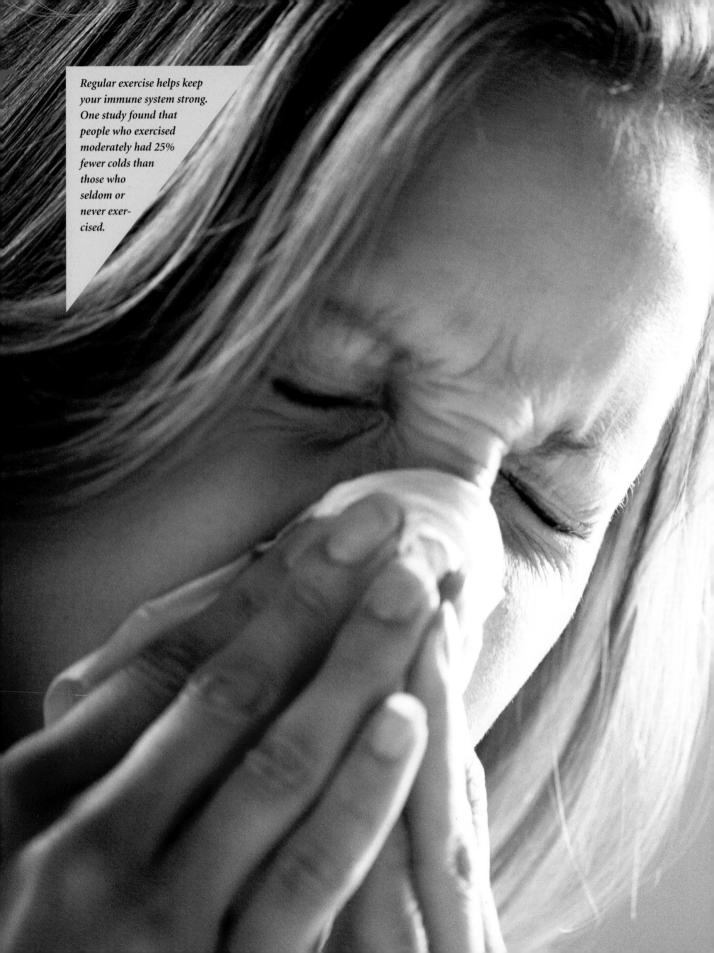

Regular exercise helps keep your immune system strong. One study found that people who exercised moderately had 25% fewer colds than those who seldom or never exercised.

How to bolster your immune system

Your body is under constant assault from invading bacteria and viruses, as well as from your own mutating cells. A healthy immune system—well-armed with white blood cells, antibodies, and certain proteins and other substances—will keep those invaders and renegades in check by destroying, devouring, or inactivating them.

Chronic stress impairs immunity. Relaxation training can help.

But a number of forces can undermine those defenses, increasing your risk of infection and possibly cancer, and slowing your recovery from illness. Weakened defenses can also give viruses that have been lurking in your system, sometimes for decades, an opportunity to pounce. For example, the virus that causes chicken pox in children can become active and cause shingles, a painful nerve disease.

You can help keep your immune system strong by eating and exercising wisely, taking certain supplements if necessary, minimizing stress, and avoiding external assaults, such as overexposure to the sun, ingestion of some pollutants, and overuse of certain medications. Those measures offer protection even in older adults, contradicting the long-held notion that immunity inevitably declines with advancing age.

Here are the details on what you can do to energize and maintain your body's defenses against disease.

FEED YOUR WHITE BLOOD CELLS

Scientists have long known that malnutrition—a grossly inadequate intake of protein and calories—can devastate the body's immune system. Now they've confirmed that insufficient intakes of certain vitamins and minerals—even moderate shortages that don't cause obvious signs of deficiency—can also undermine the body's weapons against infection and other diseases.

Nutrient shortfalls are fairly common, especially in older people who are unable to buy, prepare, and eat a balanced diet. Surveys indicate that about one-third of older people consume significantly less than the recommended amount of one or more nutrients.

The most frequently scanted nutrients include zinc, selenium, iron, the B vitamins (including folic acid), vitamins C and D, and beta-carotene. People who lack any of those tend to have signs of weakened immunity, mainly fewer and less active natural killer cells, a group of white blood cells that are the body's vital first line of defense against disease.

Supplements that may boost your immunity

Dietary supplements ranging from garlic to ginseng and melatonin, and mega-doses of various vitamins and minerals have all been promoted as boons to the immune system. While there's little if any evidence to back up most of those claims, recent research has strengthened the case for two supplements: echinacea and probiotics, or pills containing "good" bacteria, similar to those found in yogurt.

• **Echinacea.** In test-tube experiments, extracts of this herb clearly enhance the ability of various immune-system components to kill or control germs. More important, taking the herb at the first sign of a cold appears to shorten its duration and ease its symptoms by some 10 to 40 percent, according to several small clinical trials. People who have an upper-respiratory-tract infection may get a modest benefit by taking echinacea extracts or pills. However, individuals who have an autoimmune disorder such as rheumatoid arthritis, caused by an overactive immune system, should probably avoid the herb, since in theory it could worsen those conditions.

Can echinacea also prevent colds? The few clinical trials that have addressed that question have shown no clear benefit from the herb. One possible reason: Other research indicates that echinacea's immune-boosting power fades with extended use.

• **Probiotics.** Numerous studies have shown that ingesting the "good" bacteria in these pills can restore a healthy balance of organisms in the gut and activate disease-fighting antibodies there. That may help combat inflammatory bowel disease as well as diarrhea caused by infection or antibiotics. People who suffer from persistent diarrhea or are taking those medications—and have no autoimmune disorders—may want to talk with their physicians about trying a probiotic. Look for pills that contain the bacterium Lactobacillus GG or the yeast Saccharomyces boulardii, which have proved to be hardy enough to survive both the stomach's digestive acids and the antibiotic onslaught. (While some yogurts contain live bacteria, none sold in the U.S. have those particular strains.)

Other research suggests that probiotics may strengthen the functioning of the immune system throughout the body. Indeed, one study found that the pills reduced the number of potential disease-causing germs in the nasal cavity. But it's not known whether that reduction translates into protection against actual upper-respiratory-tract infections. So while the evidence is promising, it's too preliminary to warrant taking probiotics for that purpose.

Several studies have found that correcting nutritional shortages can restore normal immune function and reduce the risk of infection as well. For example, Canadian researchers found that a multivitamin/mineral supplement taken daily for one year strengthened the body's defenses and reduced the risk and duration of infection in people who had marginally low levels of various nutrients.

In well-nourished individuals, however, observational studies suggest that immune function remains relatively strong, even in most older people. Moreover, at least two clinical trials have found that taking multivitamin/mineral supplements did not lower the risk of infection in well-fed individuals.

The evidence on whether mega-doses of individual nutrients—notably vitamin E and zinc—can enhance immunity has been contradictory, especially in people who eat adequately. Indeed, a recent large clinical trial on this question found that well-nourished people who took extra vitamin E were sick longer and with worse symptoms during the 15-month study than those who took a placebo. As for extra vitamin C, there's little evidence that it helps treat colds and virtually none that it helps prevent them. ("Supplements that may boost your immunity," above, discusses two supplements that may help fortify the body's defenses.)

Recommendation: A diet rich in produce, whole grains, legumes, and low-fat dairy products should provide an ample supply of most nutrients linked to healthy immunity. People who don't consume a nutritious diet should take a daily multivitamin/mineral supplement.

But even with an ideal diet, everyone over age 50 should consume at least 2.4 micrograms per day of supplemental vitamin B12, from either fortified foods or a modest B12 or multivitamin supplement. That's because many middle-aged and older people don't produce enough stomach acid to adequately absorb that vitamin from food. While most well-fed older people's immunity does remain fairly robust, supplemental B12 can not only help ensure optimal defenses but also protect against several other potential problems caused by B12 deficiency.

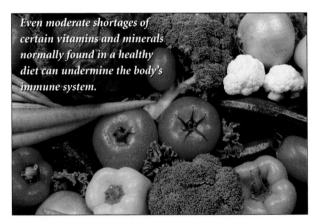

Even moderate shortages of certain vitamins and minerals normally found in a healthy diet can undermine the body's immune system.

And people who seldom get out in the sun may need supplemental vitamin D supplied by a multivitamin or a vitamin-D pill, especially if they're over age 65, when the skin's ability to synthesize the vitamin from sunlight diminishes. A daily supplement of 400 International Units (IU) of vitamin D is recommended for people in their 50s and 60s, 600 to 800 IU for older people, and 1,000 IU for people of any age who are rarely exposed to sunlight.

WORK OUT, BUT DON'T OVERWORK

During very intense exercise, the body handles the physical stress in part by pumping out the emergency hormones cortisol and adrenaline. The hormones temporarily impair immune function, which may allow viruses and bacteria to gain a foothold during those periods. That may explain why several studies have found increased susceptibility to infection among people

A diet rich in produce, whole grains, legumes, and low-fat dairy products should provide an ample supply of most nutrients linked to healthy immunity.

who exercise extremely hard—while preparing for a marathon, for example.

Workouts that aren't exhausting, however, have the opposite effect: They temporarily strengthen the immune system, by boosting the aggressiveness of natural killer cells and the bacteria-gobbling capacity of other immune cells called macrophages. Repeated often enough, those short-term boosts, lasting up to a few hours, can apparently yield substantial benefits.

Researchers at the University of South Carolina and the University of Massachusetts recently studied some 550 adults. Those who regularly exercised at least moderately had about 25 percent fewer colds during the one-year study than those who seldom or never exercised. Results of at least three small clinical trials tend to

Workouts that aren't exhausting temporarily strengthen immunity.

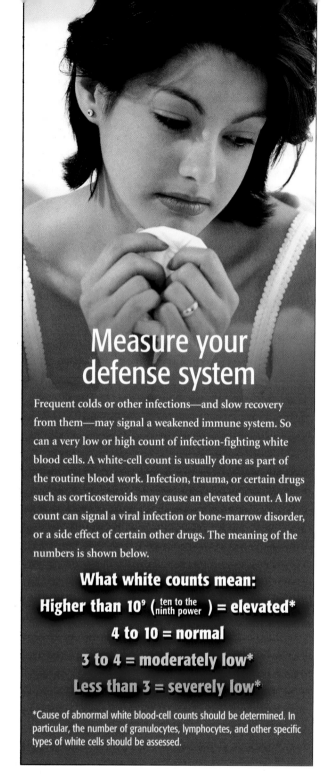

Measure your defense system

Frequent colds or other infections—and slow recovery from them—may signal a weakened immune system. So can a very low or high count of infection-fighting white blood cells. A white-cell count is usually done as part of the routine blood work. Infection, trauma, or certain drugs such as corticosteroids may cause an elevated count. A low count can signal a viral infection or bone-marrow disorder, or a side effect of certain other drugs. The meaning of the numbers is shown below.

What white counts mean:

Higher than 10^9 (ten to the ninth power) = elevated*

4 to 10 = normal

3 to 4 = moderately low*

Less than 3 = severely low*

*Cause of abnormal white blood-cell counts should be determined. In particular, the number of granulocytes, lymphocytes, and other specific types of white cells should be assessed.

---

you may find your typical workout routine exhausting, and overdoing it might undermine your battle against the bug.

If you have a more serious infection, like pneumonia or the flu—marked by fever, chills, muscle aches, fatigue, or swollen lymph glands—any exercise can overtax your struggling immune system and worsen the illness.

Recommendation: The more exercise you do, the more immune benefits you'll reap, provided you stop short of exhaustion. Avoid workouts that cause uncomfortable shortness of breath, profuse sweating in cold or

> *Research volunteers who reported the highest stress were almost twice as likely to catch a cold as those with the least stress.*

mild weather, feelings of unsteadiness, or substantial fatigue or muscle pain.

If you have a cold, ratchet down your workouts. Don't exercise at all if you have a more serious infection, and avoid intense activity for one to two weeks after symptoms disappear.

RELAX AND DEFEND

A number of studies suggest that chronic stress—whether it's caused by external pressure or internal perception—also impairs immunity. For example, researchers at Ohio State University compared people caring for a spouse who had Alzheimer's disease with other people free of that draining obligation. More than a year later, three key measures of immune function were significantly lower in the caregivers than in the others. More important, the caregivers were sick with colds for twice as many days.

In a more rigorous demonstration, researchers at Carnegie Mellon University actually sprayed a cold virus into the nostrils of some 400 volunteers. The chance of

confirm that finding. In all three, women who were told to walk briskly most days for three months developed colds only about half as often as those who didn't exercise.

Should you work out if you're already sick? When you have a cold, moderate exercise is OK if it makes you feel better. But be aware that because of your weakened state coming down with a cold was directly proportional to the volunteers' stress levels; those who reported the most tension were almost twice as likely to catch a cold as those with the least.

Steps that ease stress may improve immune function. For example, moderate exercise may boost immunity in part because it helps you relax. Preliminary research has identified several other tension tamers that may also boost immunity. Here are some examples:

• **Relaxation training.** A combination of guided imagery and self-hypnosis improved some measures of immunity in two studies of medical students; in a third, meditation alleviated the immune-dampening effect of strenuous exercise in a group of runners.

• **Social support.** People who regularly attend religious services have slightly stronger immune systems than other people, one study has found. Another study indicated that people who have a diverse and thriving network of relatives, friends, and acquaintances had a lower risk of catching cold. (Of course, that protective link is presumably weakened when your social contacts are sick.)

• **Positive attitude.** Researchers asked incoming law-school students to predict their performance and then measured their immune function during midterm exams. The most optimistic students had a more active immune system at that stressful time than their downbeat counterparts. Another study found that people who responded to stress by seeing the humor or the bright side in the situation had higher blood levels of immunoglobulin A, a key antibody, than their gloomier counterparts.

• **Massage.** Regular massages increased the number and aggressiveness of natural killer cells in one study and of disease-fighting antibodies in another.

From yoga to reading, most forms of relaxation are likely to help the immune system.

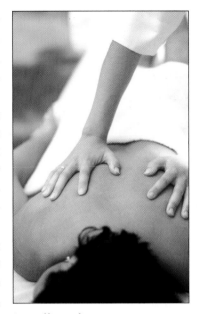

Massage can help you relax and may boost your immune system.

Recommendation: Activities that help you relax or improve your mood will likely strengthen your immunity. That includes the steps just described as well as several that haven't been adequately tested for their immune-strengthening potential, such as yoga, tai chi, progressive muscle relaxation (in which you alternately tighten and then relax your muscles), or even just reading a good book or engaging in a favorite hobby. Whichever approach you take, find some time each day to unwind.

FOUR MORE FORTIFIERS

Recent research has identified several other steps that may help bolster the immune system.

• **Get sufficient sleep.** Lack of sleep seems to cause some immune-system components to mistakenly attack the body. That may worsen autoimmune disorders such as rheumatoid arthritis and also cause arterial inflammation, which contributes to heart disease. In addition, insufficient sleep impairs the function of other immune components needed to prevent disease; in one study, a single night of partial sleep deprivation slashed the activity level of natural killer cells by about a third. And lack of sleep may be harmful in

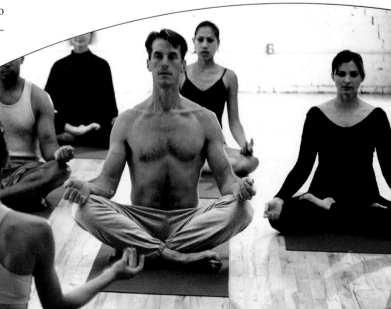

Precautions for vulnerable people

A number of diseases can severely weaken the immune system, notably certain cancers, diabetes, and HIV infection. So can certain drugs, such as corticosteroids (for inflammation) and treatments for cancer, hepatitis, and organ-transplant recipients. Anyone with severely weakened immunity is especially susceptible to potentially deadly infections and should take the following special precautions:

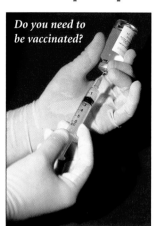

Do you need to be vaccinated?

• Get vaccinated against the flu and pneumonia. But don't get vaccinated against chicken pox, smallpox, measles, mumps, or rubella. Unlike the flu and pneumonia vaccines, those vaccines contain live viruses that can overwhelm weakened defenses.

• Practice scrupulous dental hygiene to ward off periodontal infections.

• Cook meat, fish, and eggs thoroughly to kill the bacteria that can lurk in food.

• Consider installing a water filter to extract parasites from your water.

• Apply insect repellent assiduously when outdoors, especially in the woods, to ward off infection with West Nile and Lyme diseases.

• Be especially alert to the appearance of any new symptoms, including common ones like back pain or a rash, since that could signal an underlying and potentially dangerous infection.

• Minimize hospital visits, since germs are especially plentiful and virulent there. If you're hospitalized, insist that hospital staff follow the proper precautions to prevent the spread of infection.

• Consider donating your own blood before any surgery that may require a blood transfusion, to eliminate the possibility of a blood-borne infection.

• Ask whether you should take antibiotics before undergoing periodontal work and certain major operations, notably hysterectomy and cardiac, colorectal, or joint-replacement surgery.

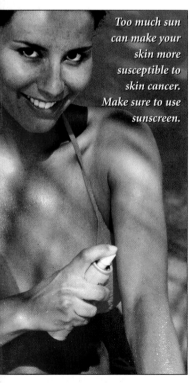

Too much sun can make your skin more susceptible to skin cancer. Make sure to use sunscreen.

other ways, too: It contributes to weight gain and diabetes by disrupting hormone levels, and it diminishes mental and physical performance.

Recommendation: Most people need seven to eight hours of sleep a night. If you sleep less than that or are often tired during the day, try to change your sleep habits. Effective strategies include establishing a regular sleep and rising time, avoiding naps, blocking out disturbances, reserving your bed only for sleep and sex, and limiting your liquid intake—especially of beverages that contain caffeine or alcohol—for a few

hours before bed. If you don't drift off to sleep within about 30 minutes, or wake up and can't fall back asleep, get up and do something quiet until you feel drowsy.

• **Avoid excessive sun exposure.** While the body needs some sunlight to produce vitamin D, too much sunshine can suppress the immune system. Overexposed skin is susceptible not only to skin cancer but also to infections, possibly because of impaired immune responses, both systemically and within the skin itself.

Recommendation: If you expect to spend more than about 20 minutes out in the sun from mid-morning to late afternoon during the warmer months in the North or year-round in the South, wear sun-protective clothing and sunglasses, and slather on sunscreen with a sun-protective factor (SPF) of at least 15.

• **Limit exposure to pesticides and mercury.** Animal and lab research suggests that those substances, especially in high doses or with extended exposure, may degrade immune function. A few observational studies have found that people who often work with mercury or certain pesticides may have weakened defenses.

Recommendation: To reduce exposure to pesticides, thoroughly wash fruits and vegetables under running water; use a soft brush and a diluted solution of dish soap to scrub apples, bell peppers, tomatoes, and other produce coated in pesticide-trapping wax. Consider buying organic produce when it's available and affordable. To minimize exposure to mercury, limit your intake of fish that may be high in the metal, such as king mackerel, shark, swordfish, and, to a lesser extent, fresh-water bass, halibut, and bluefin or canned white tuna.

Don't use antibiotics to treat viral infections, such as the common cold.

• **Limit antibiotic use.** Recent studies suggest that exposure to infection and other allergens early in life may help build a well-developed immune system. Conversely, frequent exposure to antibiotics may weaken immunity by killing the bacteria that the body would otherwise have to grapple with and that would ultimately strengthen it.

Recommendation: Don't use antibiotics to treat viral infections, such as the common cold. (The drugs won't harm the virus, but they will kill lots of the helpful bacteria that live in the body. And needless use helps breed antibiotic resistance.) Parents should also refuse antibiotic treatment for fluid buildup in their children's ears unless an examination clearly shows an infection.

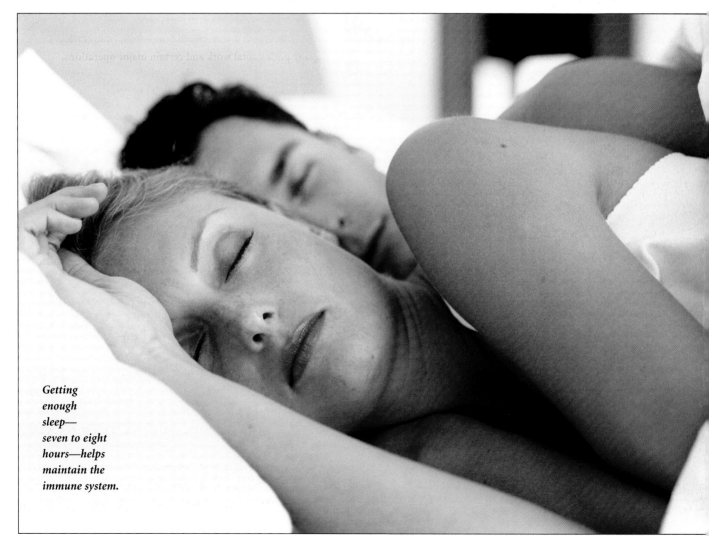

Getting enough sleep— seven to eight hours—helps maintain the immune system.

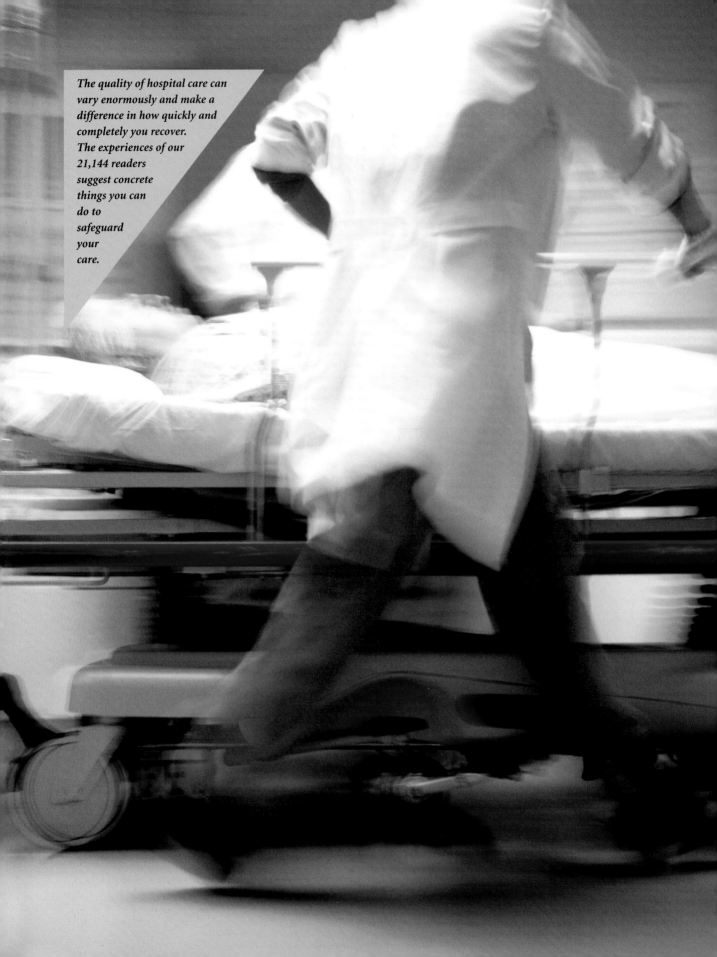

The quality of hospital care can vary enormously and make a difference in how quickly and completely you recover. The experiences of our 21,144 readers suggest concrete things you can do to safeguard your care.

How safe is your hospital?

The quality of care you receive during a hospital stay can determine how quickly and how well you recover—or if you recover at all. You might expect consistently good care to be delivered at almost every hospital in a nation with the world's top doctors,

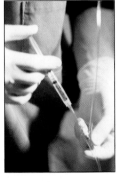

most advanced technology, and highest per-capita spending on health care. But when we surveyed and invited e-mails from CONSUMER REPORTS readers about their recent hospital experiences, we found enormous variations. They ranged from an Alabama man's smooth-sailing, life-saving, $1.5 million liver transplant to an 83-year-old Tennessee man's death after a careless emergency-room staff sent him home without treating the broken bones and internal injuries he had suffered from falling down the basement stairs.

Just how dramatically the quality of hospital care can affect your outcome was driven home to one reader, Kate Parks, from Denver, when she needed surgery twice in one month for a detached retina. Both surgeries were performed by the same doctor, but for scheduling reasons the

Play it safe: Ask the name of the medicine to double-check that you're getting the right one.

two procedures took place in different hospitals, comparable in size and facilities. At the first hospital, it took so long for anyone to answer Parks' call for assistance when she awoke after surgery that she nearly fainted while getting out of bed to use the bathroom. In contrast, after her surgery at the second hospital, a nurse not only answered her call, but also discovered the reason for Parks' lightheadedness—low blood pressure—which she treated with extra intravenous fluids. "The first time, it took me at least two or three days after I went home before I felt OK again," Parks says. "With better care the second time, I felt much better, much sooner."

Robert Brook, M.D., director of the RAND Health Institute in Santa Monica, Calif., put the matter bluntly: "Most people will just go to wherever their doctor hospitalizes them. But the hospital you're in absolutely makes a huge difference."

If, like 55 percent of our survey respondents, you have a choice of which hospital to use, this article explains the information you need to select wisely and where to find it.

Readers report on their care

Our survey, part of the CONSUMER REPORTS 2001 Annual Questionnaire, asked subscribers about hospital experiences between January 2000 and April 2001. The 5,829 people who were hospitalized for nonsurgical treatment reported less adequate care than did the 13,647 whose stay was for surgery. This is partially, but not totally, explained by the fact that a good number of surgery patients did not have an overnight stay. The 1,204 respondents who were in the hospital to have a baby had experiences similar to those of the surgical patients. Survey respondents who didn't specify the type of care they received were excluded from this analysis. These results reflect the experiences of CONSUMER REPORTS subscribers, who may not be representative of the U.S. population.

Percent who strongly agreed that...	NONSURGICAL	SURGICAL	OBSTETRICS
Staff asked regularly about pain.	44%	58%	57%
Staff treated pain adequately.	51	68	67
Nursing staff responded promptly to calls.	48	58	60
They could speak to a doctor when they wanted.	27	38	35
Staff were courteous and respectful.	66	74	70
Staffing seemed adequate to meet their needs.	52	64	66

If you don't have a choice of hospitals because you're admitted for an emergency or the hospital is dictated by your health plan or doctor, we explain how to work around problem areas to make sure you get the best possible care.

AT RISK FOR BAD CARE

A total of 21,144 readers told us about their own recent hospitalization or that of a close family member. Those who were less than highly satisfied with their hospital—22 percent—complained more often of unanswered calls for assistance, inadequate pain relief, pressure to leave the hospital too soon, or recovery prolonged by complications caused by the hospitalization.

The remaining 78 percent of respondents were highly satisfied with their stay. Overall, readers rated their hospital experiences higher than CONSUMER REPORTS survey respondents have rated service in banks, restaurants, or hotel chains in the past. But unlike most other services, the care you get at a hospital can have serious long-term consequences, so any risk of receiving substandard care must be taken seriously. Hospital studies show, for example, that your odds of dying of a heart attack or in the intensive-care unit in the worst American hospitals are two times greater than in the nation's best hospitals.

So how can you tell whether your local hospitals are up to par? The experiences of our survey respondents, together with research studies and interviews with experts across the nation, helped us to identify three crucial factors: Sufficient staff (especially registered nurses), good

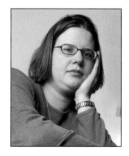

An accidental comparison

Kate Parks' back-to-back eye operations at two Denver-area hospitals were performed by the same surgeon, but her experiences were very different. At the first hospital, "very harried and uncaring nurses," she says, neglected her comfort and didn't answer her call bell in time to prevent her from nearly fainting when she got up to use the bathroom. At the second hospital, with attentive nursing care and attention to small details, like providing enough pillows, she says, "I was hugely more comfortable and felt so much better, so much sooner."

systems for organizing care, and lots of experience with your particular medical condition seem to make the most difference in both patient satisfaction and recovery.

Interestingly, the type of insurance you have does not. In our survey, the experiences of patients whose bills were paid by health maintenance organizations (HMOs) were every bit as good as those covered by fee-for-service or preferred-provider plans. The only way in which HMO patients stood out: Their out-of-pocket costs were by far the lowest.

But the type of condition for which you are admitted does affect your risk of having a bad experience. People hospitalized for nonsurgical treatment seem to be more at risk for poor care than those treated surgically or in the hospital to have a baby. In our survey, people who received nonsurgical treatment for diseases such as respiratory illness, heart failure, or cancer reported more problems with pain relief and lower satisfaction with care than did patients who had surgery.

"People who come in for surgery have an idea of what to expect, and their care is coordinated by a team," explains Susan Edgman-Levitan, P.A., a fellow at Boston's nonprofit Institute for Health Care Improvement. "In contrast, most people on medical wards are older, with complicated, multiple, chronic conditions for which there isn't a predictable course of treatment." Those patients are often treated by a doctor who doesn't know much about them and who has to wade through a foot-thick chart to find needed information.

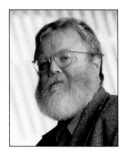

In search of pain relief

Hospitalized for a week with a serious infection following arthroscopic knee surgery, John-Michael Kramer repeatedly endured long waits for pain medication. "The nursing care was so poor, they'd take 45 minutes to an hour to show up" after he asked for pain relief, Kramer recalls. To add to his troubles, he developed a herniated disc in his back, which he blames on a sagging hospital mattress.

Patricia Seidle, who has insulin-dependent diabetes and severe heart disease, has almost come to expect uncoordinated care from the Pennsylvania hospital where she is a regular inpatient. "Every time I go in, they don't give me my insulin," she says. One time Seidle's blood sugar rose to 425 milligrams per deciliter (normal is between 60 and 110 mg/dL) before she was given insulin. Nonsurgical patients and their families need to be particularly careful to follow the recommendations below, which can help them work around hospital deficiencies.

FOR WANT OF A NURSE

Of all the factors measured in the CONSUMER REPORTS survey, satisfaction with care and attention from nurses, doctors, and other hospital staff members made the most difference by far in overall satisfaction. Moreover, only 2 percent of the survey respondents who reported attentive nursing care ended up with a serious health complication, compared with 8 percent of those who found it more difficult to get a nurse to help them.

Other evidence confirms our finding that the care that keeps patients happy also improves their health outcomes. The lower the patient-to-nurse ratio, the lower

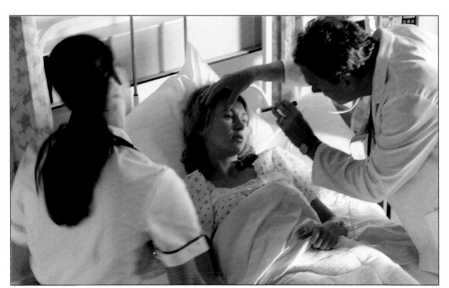

The level of care by all members of the staff can make or break a hospital stay.

the risk of common hospital-related complications, such as urinary-tract infection, pneumonia, or gastrointestinal bleeding, researchers from the Harvard School of Public Health reported recently in *The New England Journal of Medicine*. The study showed that alert nursing care made a life-or-death difference. Hospitals with ample nurse staffing had 9.4 percent fewer cases of cardiac arrest and shock than hospitals with lower staffing levels.

And the risk of death is directly related to a nurse's caseload. Every additional patient over four increases the risk of death following surgery by 7 percent, according to a study of 232,342 surgical patients in 168 Pennsylvania hospitals, published in October 2002 in the *Journal of the American Medical Association.*

But just 60 percent of our survey respondents said unequivocally that their hospital was adequately staffed, and only 55 percent strongly agreed that nurses responded promptly to calls for help.

Michelle Kellett, of Rochester, N.Y., says when her grandmother was hospitalized, "The nurses had about 14 patients each." The staff were spread so thin that nurses failed to keep a written record of one of the medications her grandmother received, and they sent her home with a bedsore on her heel so bad that she spent three extra weeks in a rehabilitation facility.

This is not an isolated incident. The shortage of nurses—particularly registered nurses—and other staff at the nation's hospitals has reached critical proportions. On average, 13 percent of nursing positions at U.S. hospitals are unfilled, with some hospitals reporting vacancy rates of more than 20 percent. And the pressures of working in understaffed units is making hospital jobs less desirable. Hospital administrators report that despite strenuous recruiting efforts, higher salaries, and sign-on bonuses of up to $10,000, they are having more and more trouble filling their nursing positions.

HOSPITAL-CAUSED ILLNESS

Even in well-staffed hospitals, care can suffer because of inefficient systems and poor communication. A 2001

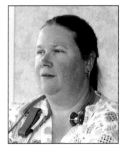

Advice from an experienced R.N.

After 18 years in nursing, Sylvia Steiger has plenty of ideas about how to improve your hospital stay. "My biggest piece of advice is to have someone with the patient to make those obnoxious demands," she says. Another tip: Bring a complete list of medications with you, including name, dose, and administration schedule. But she says the main quality variable is one patients can't control: the nurse-patient ratio.

study of health-care quality by the National Academy of Sciences said the mismatch between America's highly advanced medical technology and the chaotic system used to deliver it is "the medical equivalent of manufacturing microprocessors in a vacuum-tube factory."

The result: From 3 to 4 percent of hospital patients experience some kind of "adverse event" caused by medical error or mismanagement, major studies have found. In our survey, 12 percent of the respondents said they were aware of a medication error, misdiagnosis, or similar problem during their stay. For 5 percent of all respondents, such problems led to serious health complications.

Problems with medication delivery in hospitals have been well documented. For instance, in a study of 36 randomly selected hospitals in Georgia and Colorado, reported in the *Archives of Internal Medicine*, researchers directly observed hospital staff administering medications. They found mistakes—including staff forgetting to give the medication, giving an unauthorized drug, and giving a drug at the wrong time or in the wrong dose—in 19 percent of the doses given.

Six percent of our survey respondents reported developing an infection during or within one week of their hospital stay. Knowing a hospital's infection rate might be a good way to rate the quality of its care. But this infor-

Care that keeps patients happy also improves health outcomes.

When experience counts most

Studies of hospitals and doctors show that certain types of surgeries and medical conditions carry a significantly lower risk of mortality in facilities that see many such cases. Other surgeries don't seem to be as dependent on volume.

DIFFERENCES IN MORTALITY RISK BETWEEN LOW- AND HIGH-VOLUME HOSPITALS

SIGNIFICANT DIFFERENCE (more than 5 percent)	MODERATE DIFFERENCE (1 to 5 percent)	LITTLE DIFFERENCE (less than 1 percent)
AIDS	Colorectal-cancer surgery	Carotid endarterectomy
Esophageal-cancer surgery	Heart attack	Coronary angioplasty
Pancreatic-cancer surgery	Lung-cancer surgery	Hip-fracture repair
Pediatric heart surgery	Repair unruptured abdominal aortic aneurysm	Open-prostate removal
Repair brain aneurysm	Transurethral-prostate removal	Total hip replacement
Repair ruptured abdominal aortic aneurysm		Total knee replacement
Stomach-cancer surgery		

Source: *Annals of Internal Medicine*, Sept. 17, 2002

mation, though collected by hospitals and accrediting groups, is not released to the public.

IT STILL HURTS

Inadequate pain relief is one of the most disturbing consequences of overworked and poorly organized staff. In our survey, 37 percent of all respondents, and 49 percent of the nonsurgical patients, reported suboptimal pain relief.

John-Michael Kramer, a government consultant from Maryland, ran into both organizational and understaffing problems when he was hospitalized for a week with a knee that had become severely infected following arthroscopic surgery. Rather than receiving medication on a regular schedule, a widely recommended procedure that would have kept his agonizing pain under better control, Kramer was required to ask for every dose.

"I'd hit my call button, but the nurses would take 45 minutes to an hour to show up," he says, recalling his frustrating ordeal. "I finally hit on thetactic of calling the hospital switchboard and asking them to patch me through to the nurse's station on my ward."

Experiences such as Kramer's are the all-too-predictable result of nurse understaffing, says Patricia Rowell, R.N., senior policy fellow at the American Nurses Association. "When you're faced with a patient who wants a pain pill and another who is bleeding, the life-threatening situation is going to get attention first," Rowell says.

Better systems, such as making sure that doctors order pain medications in advance or that hospitals provide "patient-controlled analgesia" machines that enable you to safely administer your own pain medication, can reduce nursing labor and make prompt pain relief available.

"There are both medical and financial arguments in favor of treating pain," says Dennis Turk, Ph.D., a professor of anesthesiology and pain research at the University of Washington. "When their pain is well controlled, people get out of the hospital faster. When they have a lot of pain, they recover more slowly and with more complications." Yet deficiencies in pain control persist despite reform efforts and national guidelines developed by phalanxes of experts, going back two decades or more.

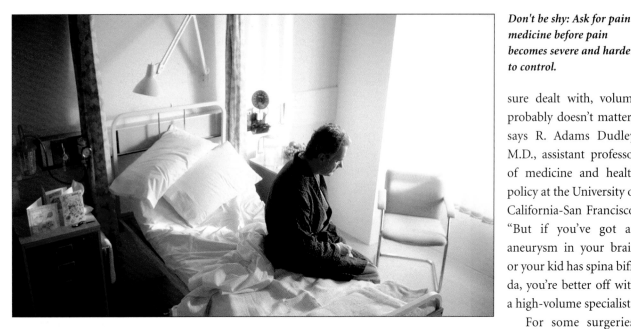

Don't be shy: Ask for pain medicine before pain becomes severe and harder to control.

THE IMPORTANCE OF EXPERIENCE

Along with good systems management and adequate staffing, the amount of experience a hospital or doctor has with a particular health condition seems to play a key role in the quality of care delivered. For many procedures and conditions, research shows that the more cases a hospital handles, the better the patients fare.

A 2002 study headed by John Birkmeyer, M.D., chief of general surgery at Dartmouth-Hitchcock Medical Center, found that the risk of death following surgery for pancreatic cancer—an especially difficult operation—is 360 percent greater at the lowest-volume hospitals than at the highest-volume ones.

In general, the experience of the hospital and surgeon are most important for uncommon, complicated, and inherently dangerous procedures, such as surgery for esophageal or pancreatic cancer, experts say. Most hospitals have plenty of experience with more common operations, such as hip replacement, breast-cancer surgery, hysterectomy, and appendectomy.

"If you're having your hernia fixed or your blood pressure dealt with, volume probably doesn't matter," says R. Adams Dudley, M.D., assistant professor of medicine and health policy at the University of California-San Francisco. "But if you've got an aneurysm in your brain or your kid has spina bifida, you're better off with a high-volume specialist."

For some surgeries, experience may not be a matter of life or death, but it still affects results. In prostate removal, for example, the mortality risk is fairly low, but the risk of bad functional outcomes, such as impotence and incontinence, seems to be

Finding an experienced hospital and surgeon is most important for uncommon and complicated procedures, such as brain aneurysm care, and less important for simpler problems like hernia repair.

lower with more experienced surgeons, notes Birkmeyer.

Fortunately, some hospital "report cards" now give consumers information on the volume of particular surgeries they perform.

RECOMMENDATIONS

The nation's $450-billion-a-year hospital industry includes some 6,000 institutions employing more than 5 million people. All too aware of its shortcomings, the industry is constantly undertaking self-improvement programs. For instance, its powerful accrediting agency, the Joint Commission on Accreditation of Healthcare

Organizations, announced in 2002 that all hospitals are required to have systems in place to prevent patient identification mix-ups and medication errors.

But you can not and should not rely on quality-improvement programs to protect you. Here are steps that patients and their family members can take to improve their chances of surviving and thriving after a hospital stay.

Make an informed choice. Among the most satisfied patients in our survey were the 20 percent who chose their hospital based on a good previous experience or because it had a good reputation. In a growing number of states and localities, it's now possible to judge hospital quality based not only on word-of-mouth but also on hard facts in publicly available hospital report cards that contain information on volume, mortality rates, and adverse outcomes.

For a list of available report cards and advice on how to use them, see "Hospital report cards" on page 122.

Just 30 of the respondents to our questionnaire said they picked their hospital based mainly on a public report card. "People aren't used to having this information, so they don't think to use it," says Judith Hibbard, Dr.P.H., a professor of health policy at the University of Oregon who is studying ways to make the report cards more useful and understandable.

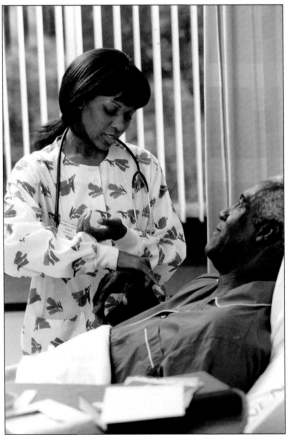

Help the hospital's busy nursing staff: Group your non-urgent requests into one call-light summons.

The bad news is that report cards aren't available in all areas. Neither is information on several of the key factors we've identified. Hospitals don't routinely measure coordination of care, adequacy of pain relief, error rates, or functional outcomes.

Hospitals know the size of their nursing staffs. But, says Patricia Rowell, senior policy fellow at the American Nurses Association, "it's sensitive information that hospitals do not wish to share." The American Hospital Association collects annual information on nurse staffing levels, but this information is available only to customers willing to purchase a costly database.

Plan ahead. Most hospitals have clinical "pathways" for various conditions, and consumers should ask for a copy, says Edgman-Levitan, of the Institute for Health Care Improvement. "Then you know what to expect, and if something doesn't happen in the right sequence, you and your family can let someone know about it," she says.

Our survey respondents were generally satisfied with the presurgical information they received. And 97 percent said the surgeon explained the surgery in a way they or their relative could understand.

Advance planning is a good way to ensure postsurgical pain relief. After suffering excruciating pain during a stay in a Texas hospital following a total knee replacement, CONSUMER REPORTS reader Mary Stark Love was determined not to have the same problem when the knee needed surgery again. "I researched pain management and talked with my surgeon about pain control, and he was totally sympathetic to my concerns," she says. The advance planning worked: Her pain stayed in check, and her recovery went much faster than after the first surgery.

Bring your own medical history. "I can't count the number of times I've admitted a patient to the hospital and asked them what meds they take, only to receive a reply like 'a blood-pressure pill in the mornings, a heart pill at dinner, and something for my arthritis,'" says Paula Estey, R.N., an Oregon intensive-care nurse.

In your wallet, carry an up-to-date list of your medication names and dosages; insurance information; names and phone numbers of your regular physicians; and key elements of your medical history, such as diabetes or a recent stroke.

Bring your own help. Patients, nurses, and national quality experts concur: Given the shortage of nurses, the most important thing to bring with you to the

Hospital staffing is so strained that those who can't fend for themselves—a child, a person under sedation, or a person who has cognitive impairment—should not be left alone unless they're in the intensive care unit.

hospital is a reliable family member or friend to run interference for you.

"No one who is basically helpless—a child, a person with a cognitive impairment, a person who cannot ambulate, a person who is sedated—should be left alone in the hospital unless they are in intensive care," says Kathleen Maynard, a Florida nurse who saw her Alzheimer's-afflicted father through four hospital stays in three years. "I am speaking as both an R.N. and a family caregiver. Hospital staffing is so strained that patients do not get the care they need."

The job of the family caregiver can range from chasing down forgotten meals to alerting someone about a worrisome symptom. For example, when Kristen Fulton's father was hospitalized for pneumonia in Ohio, she and other family members took turns staying with him. They stepped in when a nurse brought him the incorrect medication. "I don't like to think what might have happened if one of us weren't there looking after him," she says.

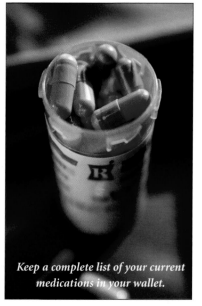
Keep a complete list of your current medications in your wallet.

Another option, elected by 2 percent of our respondents, is to hire a private-duty nurse as a "sitter" for times when family or friends can't be there. For a list of available nurses, try your hospital or local home-health-care agency. Be aware, though, that health insurance rarely covers this service.

Know the staff, and make sure they know you. Keep a list of current doctors and nurses where both you and family members can see it. If you don't recognize the health-care professional at your bedside, ask who he or she is. Also make sure all staff members check your identification bracelet before giving medication or taking you away for a test.

Write things down. Keep a notebook at your bedside, accessible to you and your family caregivers. Write down information such as medication changes, questions for the doctor and notes about his or her visit, and any significant changes in your condition. Be especially vigilant during transitions from one type of care to another—from intensive care to a regular unit, or from a hospital to a nursing home, for example. Mistakes are especially likely to occur at those times.

Double-check your medications. Ask what the medication is before you take it; if you have doubts, insist that the staff double-check the order. Sylvia Steiger, a nurse from Wyoming, says she is never insulted when a patient does this. "Usually, the doctor has changed the medication or dose, and I am able to explain that to the patient," she says. "Rarely, I have read something wrong— I'm a good nurse but far from perfect."

Be assertive about pain relief. Ask your doctor whether you are eligible for a patient-controlled analgesia machine. If you're the caregiver, don't be shy about

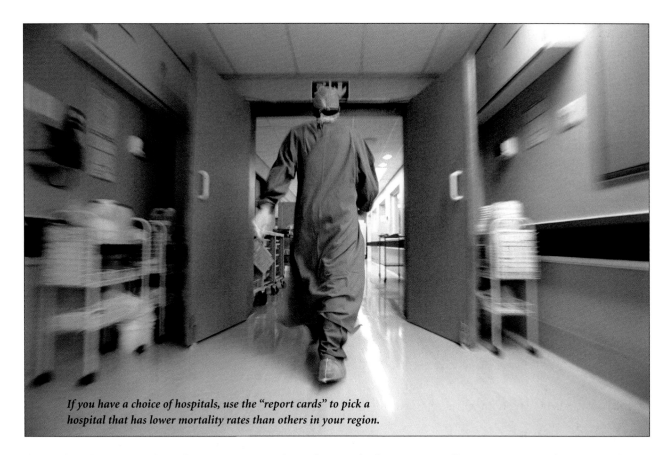

If you have a choice of hospitals, use the "report cards" to pick a hospital that has lower mortality rates than others in your region.

demanding that pain medicine be given on time; it's much more difficult to get pain under control once it has become severe. And don't forget that nonsurgical patients are often in significant pain.

Help nurses work efficiently. Find out when the hospital nursing shift changes, and try to avoid asking for anything complicated immediately after a new shift starts; nurses are especially busy then, catching up on their patients. "Batch nonurgent requests into one call-light summons," suggests Estey, the Oregon nurse. And don't be insulted if a clerk or aide responds to your call; his or her job is to separate requests that need nursing attention from those that don't.

Keep visitors under control. "Well-meaning friends and relatives simply don't realize how tiring they can be, and the patient is usually too polite to say, 'I'm exhausted, go away,'" says Steiger. Keep down the number of calls that family members make to the nursing station; designate one contact person to call for updates on the patient's condition, and organize a phone tree.

Plan your discharge. You should start preparing for discharge practically as soon as you're admitted, says Edgman-Levitan. "Start talking to the staff about what you'll be able to do when you go home and what kind of services you'll need."

Under pressure from managed care, hospitals are moving faster than ever to discharge patients as soon as they no longer need intensive hospital technology and nursing care. Seven percent of our survey respondents said the hospital tried to discharge them or their family member before they felt physically ready to leave. It pays to be assertive. About half of our respondents appealed their early discharge, and of those, two-thirds were allowed to stay longer.

Before you leave, make sure you receive a formal discharge plan from the hospital that includes provisions for follow-up care, such as doctor visits, home care, or transfer to a nursing home or rehabilitation hospital. The plan should also give explicit instructions about medication, wound care, any limits on physical activity, dietary restrictions, and which symptoms are to be expected and which are cause for concern.

Hospital report cards

The idea of hospital report cards is so new that there's no standardized way of presenting the reports or agreement on what aspects of care should be measured. User-friendliness varies widely. For those reasons, we have not rated or ranked report cards; the list below is alphabetical.

The national report cards cover the vast majority of hospitals in the U.S. The states and localities listed in the chart below are also covered by more detailed reports.

If you need surgery: Locate information for your region on volume and outcomes, such as mortality, for the surgery or procedure you are going to have. There's no standardized cut-off between good and bad hospitals, but if you have a choice, avoid hospitals whose volume numbers seem much lower or whose death rates seem much higher than others in your region. (Every report card that includes death rates has been statistically adjusted for patients' degree of illness.)

REPORT CARD	ACCESS	CONTENT	DATA SOURCES	COMMENTS
NATIONAL				
America's Best Hospitals **U.S. News & World Report**	www.usnews.com 800-436-6520 Free on Web site. List published in July, $3.95.	Ranks top 50 hospitals in each of 17 specialty areas; 177 hospitals ranked overall. Rankings based on mortality rates, available technology and services, nursing staff levels, physician survey.	Medicare records, AHA proprietary data-base, physician survey.	The only report card that contains nursing information. On the Web, searchable by hospital, location, or specialty area.
Guide to Hospitals **Consumers' Checkbook**	www.checkbook.org 800-213-7283 Print, $19.95. Free online for subscribers. Two years of Web access: $19.95 for non-subscribers.	4,500 hospitals rated. Mortality rates for 10 common medical conditions and 2 types of surgery; adverse-outcome rates for 7 types of surgery; all compared to national averages.	Medicare records, accreditation review scores, physician surveys.	Plentiful information and useful hospital safety advice. Confusing design.
Hospital Report Cards **Health Grades Inc.**	www.healthgrades.com Free for limited use. Site sells comprehensive reports on individual hospitals: $24.95 per 3 reports.	Ratings of more than 5,000 hospitals based on volume and mortality rates for 28 common procedures and diagnoses. Obstetrics data available for hospitals in 16 states, including Cesarian-section rates, volume, and complication rates.	Medicare records; for obstetrics, hospital-discharge reports.	Cumbersome search mechanism. Site only allows viewing of ratings for one procedure at a time. No overall hospital ratings.
Quality Check **Joint Commission on Accreditation of Healthcare Organizations**	www.jcaho.org Free.	Results of most-recent review by national hospital-accreditation authority. Scores for hospital services and systems compared with national results. Interactive search features.	JCAHO records.	No disease-specific or volume information.
SELECTED STATES California, Florida, Illinois, Iowa, Maryland, Massachusetts, New Jersey, New York, Pennsylvania, Virginia, Washington, Wisconsin				
Health Care Choices	www.healthcarechoices.org Free.	Volume information for specified states on high-risk cancer and cardiac surgeries. Site also links to individual state hospital-report sites.	Hospital-discharge reports.	No outcome information.
STATE HOSPITAL REPORT CARDS California, Maryland, New Jersey, New York, Pennsylvania, Texas, Virginia, Wisconsin				
CALIFORNIA California Report on Coronary Artery Bypass Graft Surgery Heart Attack Outcomes California Office of Statewide Health Planning and Development Pacific Business Group on Health	www.oshpd.state.ca.us 916-322-2814 Free.	Volume and mortality information on coronary-bypass surgery for 79 of 118 hospitals that perform it. Mortality information for 398 of 400 hospitals admitting heart-attack patients. Printed reports available.	Hospital-discharge reports.	No interactive search features. Graphs somewhat difficult to interpret

REPORT CARD	ACCESS	CONTENT	DATA SOURCES	COMMENTS
STATE HOSPITAL REPORT CARDS (cont'd)				
CALIFORNIA Patients Evaluation of Performance in California California HealthCare Foundation	www.healthscope.org 888-430-2423 Free.	Ratings of 113 California hospitals (30 percent of eligible hospitals in the state) based on patients' opinions of quality of care. Printed reports available.	Patient surveys.	Uses easy-to-follow, 1-2-3 star ratings. Can narrow online search to specific hospitals or counties. Does not measure medical outcomes.
MARYLAND Maryland Hospital Performance Evaluation Guide Maryland Health Care Commission Health Services Cost Review Commission	www.hospitalguide.mhcc state.md.us/facility_ search.asp Free.	Volume, length of stay, and readmission information for acute-care facilities 33 diagnostic groups. Information on hospital size, accreditation status. Information can be searched interactively by location or diagnosis.	Hospital-discharge reports.	Diagnostic-group terminology may be too technical to understand.
NEW JERSEY Cardiac Surgery in New Jersey New Jersey Department of Health and Senior Services	www.state.nj.us/health/ reportcards.htm 888-393-1062 Free.	Cardiac-bypass-surgery volume and mortality information for 14 hospitals and 52 individual surgeons. Can download report or order a paper copy. No interactive search features.	Hospital-discharge reports.	Clear explanation of data.
NEW YORK Cardiac Surgery Reports New York State Department of Health	www.health.state.ny.us/ nysdoh/healthinfo/inde x.htm Free.	Volume and mortality information on coronary-bypass surgery and coronary angioplasty for hospitals and individual doctors. No interactive search features.	Hospital-discharge reports.	Technical language and dense numerical tables may be difficult to understand.
PENNSYLVANIA Hospital Performance Reports Pennsylvania Health Care Cost Containment Council	www.phc4.org 717-232-6787 Free.	Vast site with volume, mortality, length-of-stay, and other outcome information for 75 diagnostic groups. Separate, more-detailed reports on coronary-bypass surgery, heart-attack care, and Cesarian-section rates. Information can be searched interactively. Regional reports can be downloaded or ordered in printed version.	Hospital-discharge reports.	Amount of information can be overwhelming. Coronary-bypass-surgery volume and outcome information available on individual physicians as well as hospitals.
TEXAS Indicators of Inpatient Care in Texas Hospitals Texas Health Care Information Council	www.thcic.state.tx.us 512-482-3312 Free.	Volume and mortality information for 25 procedures and conditions; frequency information for selected procedures, including Cesarian section and laproscopic gall-bladder surgery. Can view reports as detailed tables or bar graphs	Hospital-discharge reports.	Web site difficult to navigate, but report graphs easy to understand. Site includes useful explanatory information.
VIRGINIA Cardiac Care Virginia Health Information	www.vhi.org 877-844-4636 Free.	Volume information for 39 diagnostic groups. Volume and mortality rates for open-heart surgery, invasive cardiology, and medical cardiology.	Hospital-discharge reports.	Sponsoring group also sells information to businesses.
SOUTH-CENTRAL WISCONSIN QualityCounts Employer Health Care Alliance Cooperative	www.qualitycounts.org 608-276-6620 or 800-223-4139 Free.	Quality ratings of overall surgical and medical care, hip and knee surgery, cardiac care, and maternity care at 24 hospitals contracting with the sponsoring employer alliance.	Hospital-discharge reports.	Easy-to-understand ratings chart. Based on mortality and complication rates. No information on volume of services delivered.

When acupuncture may help

Studies show that acupuncture may be effective in relieving nausea and dental and arthritic pain.

Today's medical journals are teeming with positive anecdotes about acupuncture. Just since 2002, doctors have published almost 100 case reports in which the ancient Chinese treatment improved everything from hiccups to insomnia to prostate symptoms. But individual success stories cannot predict how well acupuncture will work in the average individual; only clinical trials can do that.

So what do those trials tell us about the benefits of acupuncture? They suggest that it may be effective for relieving certain types of pain and nausea. But clinical-trial results have been either inconclusive or negative for a host of other conditions, including asthma, back and neck pain, fibromyalgia (a chronic, painful musculoskeletal disorder), infertility, and irritable bowel syndrome; and for such uses as inducing labor and smoking cessation.

Even evidence for the use of acupuncture must often be interpreted with caution. That's because many studies have not used a convincing control treatment to rule out the placebo effect. However, some studies have used an effective control, called sham needling, in which researchers insert needles at random points that aren't supposed to be effective.

Overall, the best studies suggest that acupuncture may be worth trying for the following conditions:

• **Dental pain.** Studies have consistently shown that acupuncture is superior to control treatments—including sham needling—in the dentist's office. The evidence is especially strong for blunting postoperative dental pain, according to a 1997 National Institutes of Health consensus panel on acupuncture.

• **Nausea and vomiting.** Five of the seven clinical trials with sham-needle controls have shown that acupuncture helps keep nausea and vomiting at bay after surgery or chemotherapy. One review of the evidence concluded that needle treatment may be equivalent to medication in preventing postoperative nausea and vomiting.

• **Arthritic pain.** Needles might help relieve the discomfort of osteoarthritic knees but probably won't improve their function. That's the conclusion of a review, published in *Arthritis and Rheumatism* in 2001, of seven controlled clinical trials, including three with sham needling, involving some 400 patients. Evidence of acupuncture's benefits for rheumatoid arthritis is far weaker, another review concluded.

• **Headache pain.** In early 2004 the Cochrane Collaboration, a respected British research organization, published an evaluation of 14 clinical trials with sham-needle controls involving more than 400 migraine or tension-headache sufferers. Those trials tend to support the notion that acupuncture eases headache pain, but more convincing evidence is needed, the report concluded. So while acupuncture might help, don't toss your pain drugs just yet.

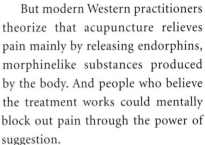

Acupuncture needles cause little or no pain; adverse reactions are rare.

HOW IT WORKS

The traditional Chinese view is that health is governed by opposing yin (spirit) and yang (blood) forces, which flow through body channels called meridians. Unbalanced forces are said to cause illness. Needles placed at prescribed spots along the meridians are believed to stimulate the flow of qi, or healing energy, and thus restore balance.

But modern Western practitioners theorize that acupuncture relieves pain mainly by releasing endorphins, morphinelike substances produced by the body. And people who believe the treatment works could mentally block out pain through the power of suggestion.

Acupuncture needles cause little or no pain, and adverse reactions are rare. Infections are the most serious, so make sure your provider uses only sterile, disposable needles. People with pacemakers should avoid acupuncture techniques that use electrical stimulation. And those who take blood thinners or have bleeding disorders should probably shun the needles.

Before trying acupuncture, have your doctor diagnose your condition, and try conventional treatments shown to be effective. If they don't help you, and there's evidence that acupuncture may provide relief, see "How to find an acupuncturist," below.

How to find an acupuncturist

The American Academy of Medical Acupuncture (800-521-2262; *www.medicalacupuncture.org*) lists medical doctors with more than 200 hours of special training. The National Certification Commission for Acupuncture and Oriental Medicine (703-548-9004; *www.nccaom.org*) certifies M.D. and non-M.D. practitioners who have had at least three years of training and have passed a test. Treatment typically costs $75 to $150 for the first visit, $35 to $75 afterward. Insurers are more likely to reimburse you if a doctor refers you for acupuncture or actually performs the treatment.

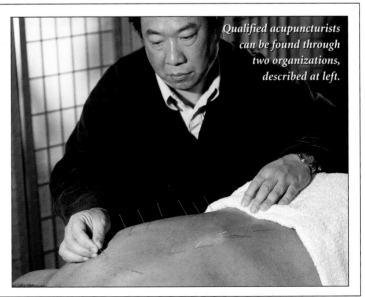

Qualified acupuncturists can be found through two organizations, described at left.

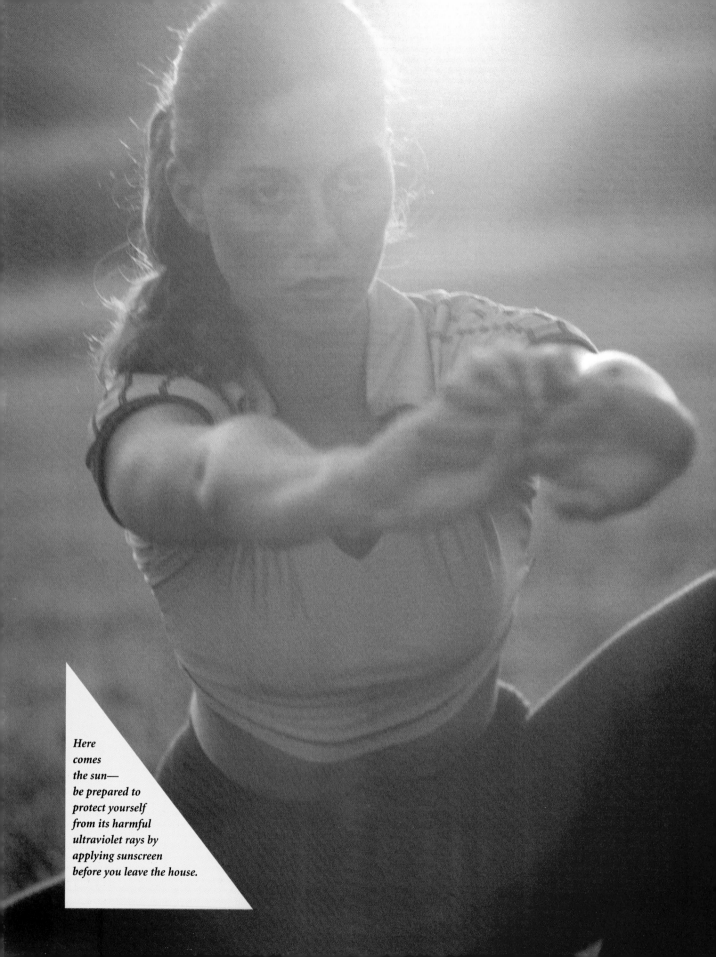

Here comes the sun— be prepared to protect yourself from its harmful ultraviolet rays by applying sunscreen before you leave the house.

Block that sun

Old-fashioned methods, such as a wide-brimmed hat and sunglasses, help protect your face.

M ore than two decades ago manufacturers introduced potent sunscreens designed to block most of the sun's damaging ultraviolet rays. Yet the ad campaigns and public-health messages about slathering on sunscreen have not yet had any apparent impact on cancer risk.

The rates of basal-cell and squamous-cell carcinomas (the most common types of skin cancer) and of melanoma (the deadliest type) have all been rising steadily. One study has even suggested that sunscreen use may increase the risk of melanoma—perhaps by creating a false sense of security about prolonged sun exposure.

Scientists have little doubt that correct use of sunscreen does protect the skin from damage. But sunscreen users may overrely on that protection. An American Cancer Society survey of adolescents found that more than one-third had been wearing sunscreen with a sun protection factor (SPF) of at least 15 when they experienced their worst sunburn of the summer.

While about half of Americans don't use a sunscreen in the summer, others may become so sun-shy that they could suffer harm from too little sun. Sunlight stimulates the skin to make vitamin D, which helps maintain bone strength and may possibly cut the risk of arthritis and even cancer. While younger people generally don't need to worry about underexposure, the skin's ability to make the vitamin declines with age. So people over age 50 need to get some unscreened sun exposure. Fortunately, it doesn't take much.

Virtually everyone can avoid health hazards and enjoy the outdoors by striking the right balance between sun and shade. Today's safe-sun approach involves brief unscreened exposure if necessary, correct sunscreen use, protective clothing, sunglasses, and common sense.

SUNSCREEN SENSE

Sunscreens help protect the skin against a type of ultraviolet radiation called UVB, which causes sunburn and skin cancer. Some sunscreens also protect against UVA radiation, which is also linked with skin cancer as well as with aging of the skin and drug-related skin reactions.

Sunscreen use is not as controversial as some reports might lead you to believe. It's true that a 1998 review of ten studies found little evidence that sunscreens protect against melanoma. And a study published that same year in the *Journal of the National Cancer Institute* found an apparent link between sunscreen use and increased risk of pre-melanoma skin growths. But the institute's Maria Turner, M.D., and many other experts believe those findings may be largely explained by people's apparent tendency to stay out in the sun longer than usual after applying sunscreen.

In theory a product with an SPF of 15 lets you stay in the sun 15 times longer than usual without burning. But research shows that people typically apply sunscreen far too thinly or unevenly. So people who think they can safely lie out in the sun all day because a sunscreen label says "SPF 15" may actually be getting only one-fourth to one-half of that protection.

The truth is that sunscreen can protect against sunburn—and may yet prove to protect against skin cancer—provided you choose the right product and use it properly. To help consumers compare over-the-counter sunscreens, including makeup containing sunscreen, the Food and Drug Administration in 2002 enacted new guidelines on label claims. The FDA banned absolute claims such as "waterproof," "all-day protection," and "sunblock," which may give people a false sense of security. However, the agency allows "water resistant" and "very water resistant" claims.

Further, manufacturers must not only list the product's SPF but also label it as providing minimum, moderate, or high sun protection. SPFs higher than 30 will be listed as "30 plus" because the agency thinks they offer little additional benefit compared with an SPF of 30, and they may expose people to needlessly high levels of chemicals.

Considering the new labels on sunscreens, Consumers Union's medical consultants recommend these steps when choosing a sunscreen:

Choose the right number. Look for the least expensive sunscreen labeled SPF 15 or more. (Most SPF 15 sunscreens we've tested lived up to the protection their labels pledged.) Even dark-skinned people should use a sunscreen of at least 15. While dark skin does seem to provide protection, especially against melanoma, overexposure can still cause burning, skin aging, and other skin cancers.

High-risk individuals should look for a product labeled SPF 30. Those individuals include people who have fair skin, lots of moles, a family history of melanoma, or a personal history of any skin cancer; or who take a drug that increases sensitivity to the sun (see "Drug-sun interactions," on the opposite page).

Seek broad coverage. Choose products that screen both UVA and UVB: those that say so on the label or that contain titanium dioxide, zinc oxide, or avobenzone.

Apply with care. Shake the container well to mix the ingredients. If you'll be scantily dressed, use at least an ounce—a generous handful—to carefully cover all exposed areas. Don't forget about your ears, which are hot spots for cancer.

Bring your watch. Even if you're wearing a sunscreen, limit your time in the summer sun to about one to three hours at midday at the most, depending on your skin type and history, the latitude, the strength of the sunscreen, how carefully you've applied it, and how much you've sweated.

Reapply when wet. If you've been sweating a lot, apply more sunscreen; reapply it immediately if you've been in the water. (However, repeat applications do not prolong the time you can safely stay in the sun.) Sunscreens currently labeled "waterproof" generally do resist being washed off better than other products. So you may want to choose such a sunscreen if you spend a lot of time in the water, which the sun does penetrate. Even waterproof sunscreen should be reapplied after swimming, since much of it may be toweled off.

Note that beach umbrellas protect you from only 40 to 50 percent of the sun's radiation; the rest reaches you from reflection off the sand and sky. Similarly, don't be fooled by overcast skies: Anywhere from 10 to 50 percent of the ultraviolet radiation penetrates the clouds. So if you'll be outside for

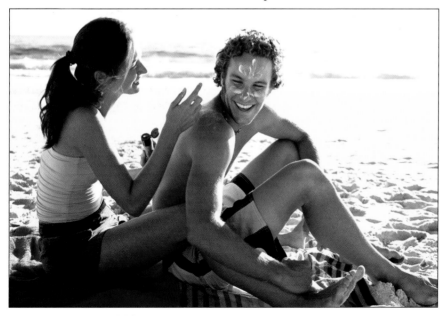

Numbers game: Choose a sunscreen with an SPF of at least 30 if you're at high risk for skin cancer.

Drug-sun interactions

A surprising number of prescription drugs can increase sensitivity to ultraviolet radiation in sunlight, causing sunburns, rashes, and other skin reactions. The table at right lists some of the more commonly used medications that can trigger such photosensitivity reactions. If you use any of these drugs, safeguard yourself by trying to avoid direct exposure to the sun and by scrupulously following the protective steps described in the main story, including use of sunscreen, protective clothing, and sunglasses.

Used for	Medication	Common brands
Acne or aging skin	Tretinoin	Avita, Renova, Retin-A
Allergies	Promethazine	Phenergan
Arthritis	Naproxen	Naprosyn
	Piroxicam	Feldene
Bacterial infection	Ciprofloxacin	Cipro
	Doxycycline	Vibramycin
	Minocycline	Minocin
	Sulfamethoxazole and trimethoprim	Bactrim
	Tetracycline	Achromycin
Depression	Doxepin	Sinequan
Diabetes	Chlorpropamide	Diabinese
Hypertension or heart failure	Chlorothiazide	Diuril
	Hydrochlorothiazide	HydroDiuril
Irregular heartbeat	Amiodarone	Cordarone
Nausea	Prochlorperazine	Compazine
Psoriasis	Methoxsalen	8-MOP, Oxsoralen
Psychosis	Chlorpromazine	Thorazine

Chart originally appeared in the July 2000 issue of CONSUMER REPORTS.

any length of time on a cloudy day or under a beach umbrella, you still need to take sunscreen and clothing precautions. And don't rely on cooler temperatures: Given the same season, time of day, and sky conditions, you'll burn just as fast when it's 70° F as when it's 90°.

Get a *little* exposure. People over age 50 or so do need to ensure an adequate supply of vitamin D, preferably by exposing their unscreened skin briefly to the sun as well as by consuming foods rich in vitamin D, such as fortified milk and fatty fish. On average, about five to ten minutes of exposure to the face, hands, and arms, two or three times a week during the summer months, will let your body store up an ample supply of vitamin D for the entire year. People who have dark skin or live in Northern latitudes need somewhat more exposure, while those who live in the South or have fair skin need less. Older people who rarely get out in the sun or seldom drink milk should take a modest vitamin-D supplement, containing 400 IU (international units) to at most 1,000 IU.

DRESS FOR THE SUN

High-risk individuals and anyone else who wants plenty of protection should wear sun-shielding apparel in warm weather, at least during the midday hours. In addition to long sleeves and long pants or skirts, two features of the cover-up outfit deserve special comment:

Cap it off. People who are at high risk or who spend a lot of time in the sun should protect their eyes, scalp, ears, and neck by wearing a hat with at least a 3-inch brim all the way around.

Watch the weave. You could get too much sun even when fully clothed if you're wearing fabric that's too porous. Here's a simple test: Any fabric that lets you see pinpoints of light when it's held up to strong illumination may have an insufficient SPF.

Fabric brighteners found in many laundry detergents absorb UV radiation, so washing clothes with them can boost a fabric's sun-shielding ability. In addition, darker fabrics absorb more light, including UV radiation. They may feel warmer, but they may also provide more protection.

Protect your eyes. Sunlight, especially UVB, contributes to the development of cataracts, vision-clouding clumps in the lens of the eye. So it's a good idea for everyone to wear sunglasses, at least during the warmer months.

Disease-fighting B vitamins

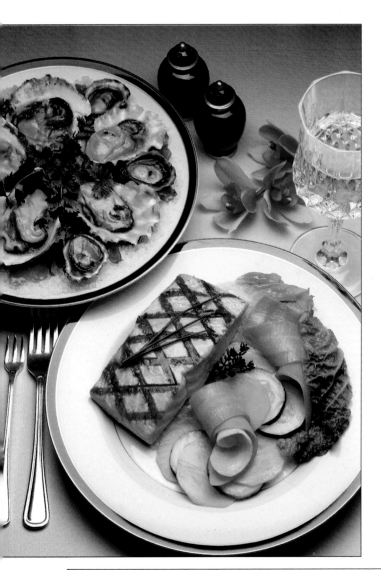

Most Americans don't get enough of the crucial B vitamins—folate (folic acid), B12, and B6—in their diet, according to the latest government data. That's partly because getting enough B vitamins can be problematic for middle-aged and older people, pregnant women, and vegetarians.

A growing body of research indicates that folate, B12, and B6 may help prevent heart disease and other serious problems, in part by lowering blood levels of the harmful amino acid homocysteine. Here are the facts about homocysteine and the three B's—and the best dietary sources of those key nutrients.

THE BENEFICIAL B'S

Homocysteine can damage the blood vessels that nourish the heart and the brain. A recent analysis of 72 studies concluded that very high levels of homocysteine not only predict heart attack and stroke but probably help cause them as well. Moreover, the long-running Framingham Heart Study found that people with an elevated homocysteine level (greater than 14 micromoles/liter) had nearly double the risk of developing Alzheimer's disease.

It's too early to recommend routine homocysteine testing for everyone. But consider asking about the test if you have a personal or family history of coronary disease

Shellfish and salmon are just two of the many foods that are high in B vitamins.

but none of the usual risk factors (smoking, excess weight, high blood pressure, high cholesterol), or if you have standard risk factors but it's unclear how aggressively to treat them.

To reduce elevated homocysteine, doctors are increasingly prescribing high doses of folic acid, though as yet there's no conclusive evidence that such supplementation actually reduces cardiovascular risk. High intakes of folate (more than 1,000 micrograms a day from all sources) can mask deficiency of vitamin B12 by correcting the anemia that often signals the problem. So people taking folic acid to lower homocysteine should first be tested for B12 deficiency, and they should consume extra B12 along with extra folate.

Whether or not you know your homocysteine level, it's wise to try keeping it down by consuming enough of all three B vitamins, preferably from food. Observational studies have linked the vitamins themselves to reduced risk of cardiovascular and Alzheimer's disease. And getting your B's can do more than just lower homocysteine. Since 1998, the U.S. government has required that all enriched-grain products be fortified with folic acid to help prevent serious birth defects. In addition, B12 seems to have an independent effect on cognitive and nerve function; large deficiencies can produce dementia, depression, or serious nerve problems. And insufficient B12 or folate can cause anemia.

DO YOU NEED A SUPPLEMENT?

Most relatively young adults should be able to get enough of the three B vitamins from foods—provided they choose the right ones (see table at right). But certain groups need supplementation:

• Adults over age 50, who may no longer produce enough stomach acid to extract vitamin B12 from food sources, should consume extra B12 from fortified foods, a multivitamin, or a modest 3- to 6-micrograms daily supplement.

• Pregnant women or women planning to become pregnant should be sure to take a prenatal vitamin to help prevent neural tube defects in the fetus.

• Vegetarians should follow the same B12 guidelines as adults over 50, since most natural sources of B12 are animal-derived. Or they should consume adequate B12 alternatives, such as certain types of nutritional yeast.

Where the B's are

KEY:
● 0-9% of DV ● 10-19% of DV ● 20-29% of DV ● 30% or more of DV

FOOD	FOLATE	B12	B6
Meat and seafood (3 oz)			
Alaskan king crab	●	●	●
Atlantic salmon	●	●	●
Beef, top round	●	●	●
Blue mussels	●	●	●
Bluefin tuna	●	●	●
Chicken breast, no skin	●	●	●
Chicken liver	●	●	●
Clams	●	●	●
Ground beef, extra lean	●	●	●
Leg of lamb	●	●	●
Lobster	●	●	●
Sardines	●	●	●
Fruits and vegetables*			
Asparagus (1/2 cup)	●	●	●
Avocado (1)	●	●	●
Banana (1)	●	●	●
Broccoli (1/2 cup)	●	●	●
Orange juice, fresh (1 cup)	●	●	●
Potato, baked with skin	●	●	●
Spinach (1/2 cup)	●	●	●
Watermelon (1 slice)	●	●	●
Dairy			
Milk, skim (1 cup)	●	●	●
Yogurt, nonfat plain (1 cup)	●	●	●
Legumes (1/2 cup)*			
Black-eyed peas	●	●	●
Garbanzo beans	●	●	●
Lentils	●	●	●
Pinto beans	●	●	●
Grains, nuts, and seeds**			
Peanuts (1/4 cup)	●	●	●
Rice, white (1/2 cup cooked)	●	●	●
Spaghetti (1/2 cup cooked)	●	●	●
Sunflower seeds (1/4 cup)	●	●	●
Wheat germ, toasted (1/4 cup)	●	●	●
Miscellaneous			
Nutritional yeast (1 tbsp)	●	●	●

Note: The FDA's recommended Daily Values (DV) are folate (folic acid), 400 micrograms; vitamin B12, 6 micrograms; vitamin B6, 2 milligrams.
*All vegetables and legumes cooked.
**Values include folic-acid fortification where applicable.
Chart originally appeared in the January 2004 issue of CONSUMER REPORTS on Health newsletter.

Water, salt,

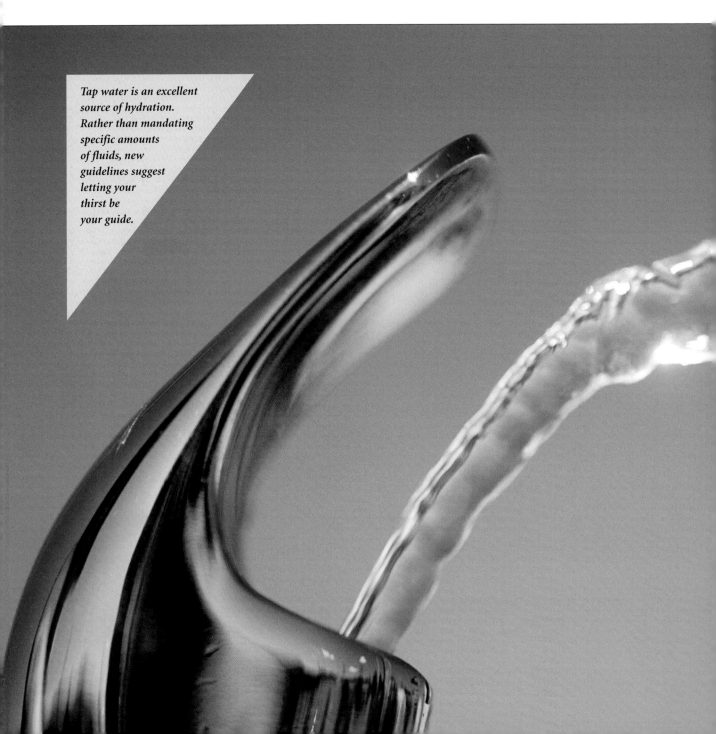

Tap water is an excellent source of hydration. Rather than mandating specific amounts of fluids, new guidelines suggest letting your thirst be your guide.

potassium:

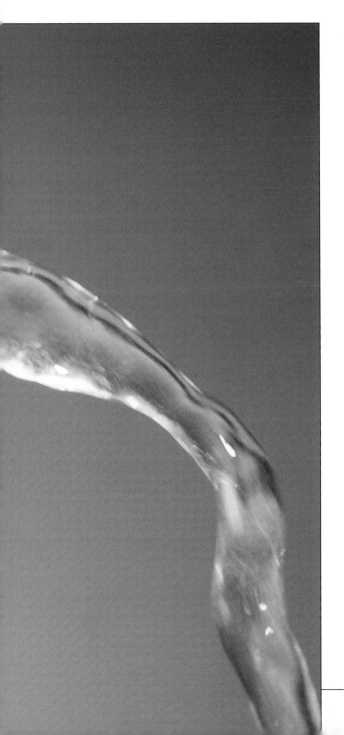

How much is enough?

Nearly three-quarters of Americans know that experts recommend drinking eight glasses of water a day, though about half admit to drinking less, according to a survey sponsored by the International Bottled Water Association. But there's good news for those who don't want to count what they drink. Americans are not suffering from a water deficit, according to a 2004 report by a panel of experts convened by the National Academy of Sciences' Institute of Medicine, which advises the government about recommended levels of nutrients.

After reviewing more than 400 studies, panel members rejected the conventional wisdom regarding water consumption. They also established new standards for the intake of sodium, potassium, and other electrolytes, the minerals that reflect the adequacy of the body's hydration.

The typical American diet is deficient in potassium and laden with too much salt, panel members concluded.

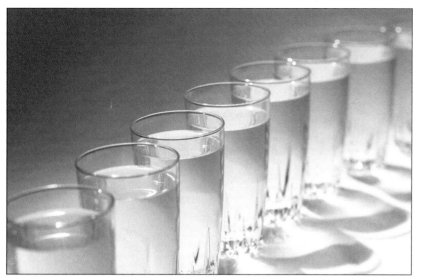

They recommended lowered levels of sodium intake, a change that may encourage the food industry to reformulate oversalted products.

So, are you drinking enough? Getting the right amount of minerals? We've waded through the data and talked to the experts to answer your questions about how these guidelines can help you stay healthy.

Should I still drink six to eight glasses of water a day?

When IOM panel members looked at studies of serum osmolality, a measure of fluid deficit or overload, they concluded that most people stay sufficiently hydrated simply by following their customary eating and drinking routines.

The origin of the eight-glasses-a-day rule is most likely government guidelines from the 1940s that recommended "1 milliliter of water for each calorie of food," or roughly 64 to 80 ounces per day. However, "water" referred to the total fluid intake from all beverages and food.

The new guidelines reflect a trend toward increased fluid consumption in the American diet but don't provide a one-size-fits-all recommendation for fluid intake. As a rough measure, the panel set the midpoint of the range of U.S. water consumption as the level that's assumed adequate for most people. For men, that's about 15½ eight-ounce cups of total water (about 13 cups from water and other beverages); for women, 11½ cups (about 9 cups from fluids).

You need to pay special attention to your fluid intake when you're active, the temperature exceeds 80° F, the humidity is low, or you're at elevations above 5,000 feet. Under these conditions more water is lost through breathing and perspiration. Most people will find themselves extra thirsty during and after such stresses, so over the course of the day, following your natural inclination should still allow you to take care of your water needs.

Do older people need to drink more?

No. The IOM recommendations for fluid intake are the same for all adults. A recent study conducted by geriatric and nutrition researchers from across the U.S. and England rejects the notion that older people should be encouraged to drink more because of chronic dehydration. Using accurate measurements of fluid intake and urine output in 450 people ages 40 to 79, the researchers found that people of all ages vary widely in their intake, but the oldest group was as well-hydrated as the youngest.

The sense of thirst diminishes with age, increasing older people's risk of dehydration from heat or exercise.

However, the sense of thirst does tend to diminish with age, increasing older people's risk of dehydration from heat or exercise. So they should be careful to drink a cup of water before and after exercise, plus another 4 ounces every 20 minutes or so during workouts—more if they're strenuous or in the heat.

How can I tell if I'm drinking enough?

The simplest way is to check your urine. Scanty, strong-smelling, dark urine is a signal that you need to drink more. Color alone is not a good indicator because medications, vitamins, and diet can all affect color.

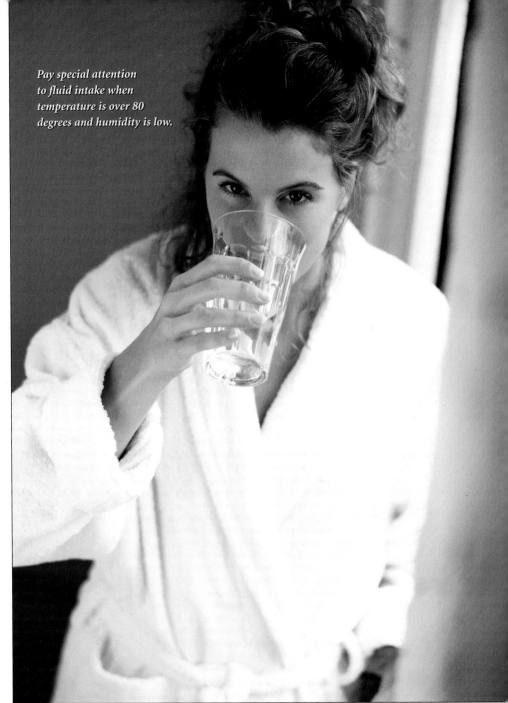

Pay special attention to fluid intake when temperature is over 80 degrees and humidity is low.

Do I have to drink plain water?

No. The IOM panel concluded that all fluids—including soft drinks, caffeinated beverages, and alcoholic drinks—factor into your daily water totals.

Caffeine earned its reputation as a diuretic from small, short-term studies of people who consumed higher doses than normal or who weren't used to drinking it. When researchers studied caffeine in men who were used to drinking it, they found no diuretic effect. Evidence on alcohol is scant but suggests that one or two drinks have no overall diuretic effect.

Plain tap water has its advantages: It's cheap, thirst quenching, and calorie free. If you dislike the taste of tap water, try bottled water. One study found that flavored waters help some people drink more and stay better hydrated. Other choices include iced tea and mixes of juice and water.

Can drinking a lot help with weight loss?

There's no scientific evidence that it can. According to Barbara Rolls, Ph.D., professor of nutritional sciences at Pennsylvania State University, water empties from the stomach very quickly and has little effect on appetite. However, studies show that eating foods with higher water content—such as fruits, vegetables, soups, and cooked grains—makes people feel fuller and less hungry than eating drier foods and drinking water with them.

Can you drink too much water?

It's possible, but not likely in healthy people who let their thirst guide them. If your body retains water because of congestive heart failure, hypothyroidism, or long-term use of certain medications—notably non-steroidal anti-inflammatory drugs such as ibuprofen, ketoprofen, and naproxen—you need to be careful not to exceed recommended fluid intakes. When you overhydrate, sodium concentrations can drop precipitously low, allowing water to leak into brain cells, causing headache, confusion, personality changes, and even seizures, coma, or death.

In the last few years athletes—particularly amateurs competing in marathons and other endurance events—who take too literally the common advice to "drink as much as possible" have emerged as another risk group. To prevent overhydration, exercisers should make sure fluid consumption stays within the range of about 1½ cups to 3 cups an hour.

What about drinking plenty of fluids when you're sick?

There's actually no scientific support for drinking more than usual, and at least theoretical reasons it could do harm. People with a lower-respiratory infection, such as pneumonia or bronchitis, may secrete an antidiuretic hormone that, along with increased fluid intake, could lead to water overload. In theory the same thing could happen during an upper-respiratory infection, such as the common cold or the flu.

To play it safe, don't drink more than a cup or so per hour.

Do I need to watch my sodium intake?

If you're like most Americans, probably yes. Sodium, which comes mainly from salt, is essential to health, but most of us get much more than we need. The new IOM guidelines define a range of daily sodium intakes, with 1,500 milligrams (mg) deemed adequate for good health (less for older people) and 2,300 mg the maximum you can consume without possibly increasing your risk of high blood pressure, particularly if you have risk factors (see next question).

Unfortunately, more than 75 percent of sodium comes from processed and restaurant foods, so reducing intake to the 1,500-mg level requires making almost all meals at home, from scratch. Even the 2,300-mg upper limit isn't easy to maintain; only about 25 percent of American women and almost no men come close to staying below it.

For many people, ingesting too much sodium could lead to high blood pressure—a serious risk factor in heart disease and stroke. Some studies suggest a link between high sodium intake and other diseases, such as stomach cancer and the worsening of asthma. And because sodium increases the excretion of calcium into the urine, it could increase bone loss and the risk of kidney stones.

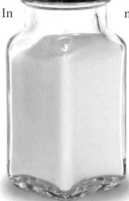

The typical American diet includes too much salt, mostly from processed and restaurant foods.

Will a low-sodium diet protect my heart?

It's clearly worth a try if you have blood pressure above the optimal limit for normal, 120/80 millimeters of mercury (mm Hg), or risk factors for hypertension. For other people, moderate sodium restriction is a more realistic goal.

Evidence for the revised recommendations comes from a government-funded trial known as the Dietary Approaches to Stop Hypertension (DASH) study, which found that cutting sodium to 1,500 mg lowers nearly everyone's blood pressure. Although the effect was slight in those with normal blood pressure, the low-sodium diet reduced systolic blood pressure (the upper number) by 3 to 7 mm Hg in those with high blood pressure or risk factors for it. Those factors include being older or black, having a family history of high blood pressure, or having high-normal blood pressure.

The benefits of sodium restriction were especially striking when combined with the DASH diet—a diet high in fruits, vegetables, whole grains, and low-fat dairy products. Those who consumed the least sodium along with the DASH diet dropped their systolic pressure by an average of 11.5 mm Hg.

For people with normal blood pressure and no risk factors, the more modest goal of 2,300 mg, achievable by adopting the DASH diet alone, would presumably help fight the upward creep in pressure that tends to occur with age.

Because some people respond dramatically to sodium, even those with high blood pressure don't necessarily have to make it all the way down to 1,500 mg to see a meaningful decline, although the less sodium consumed, the lower blood pressure will likely go. Conversely, not everyone responds to a low-sodium diet. So if you give it several months of serious effort and see no improvement, you can ease up on severe restrictions.

What are the risks of potassium deficiency?

Although severe potassium deficiency is rare, moderate deficiency is quite common and is associated with increased blood pressure, salt sensitivity, and risk of muscle weakness, kidney stones, and bone loss. Observational data suggest that it may also increase the risk of cardiovascular disease, particularly stroke.

IOM panel members found the case for potassium so compelling that they raised the recommendations from 3,500 mg per day to 4,700 mg. Unfortunately, Americans currently consume far less than that amount. Multiple daily servings of fruit, vegetables, and dairy products are the best sources of potassium.

The IOM panel said it was plausible that people taking diuretics that decrease potassium levels would need more than 4,700 mg, but the data are lacking. However, there are potassium-sparing diuretics on the market, such as amiloride (Midamor) and spironolactone (Aldactone).

Would increasing my potassium intake help my high blood pressure?

Yes. It's likely to reduce both systolic and diastolic pressure by a few points each. Potassium appears to blunt the blood-pressure-raising effects of salt, at least in part by causing the body to excrete more sodium into the urine.

Some medical conditions and medications interfere with the body's ability to excrete excess potassium. Before substantially increasing your potassium intake, check with your doctor if you have diabetes, kidney disease, heart failure, or an adrenal-gland disorder, or if you take any of the following medications: ACE inhibitors, potassium-sparing diuretics, or angiotensin receptor blockers (ARBs), such as losartan (Cozaar) and valsartan (Diovan).

Healthy combo: restricted use of salt when cooking at home and adopting the DASH diet.

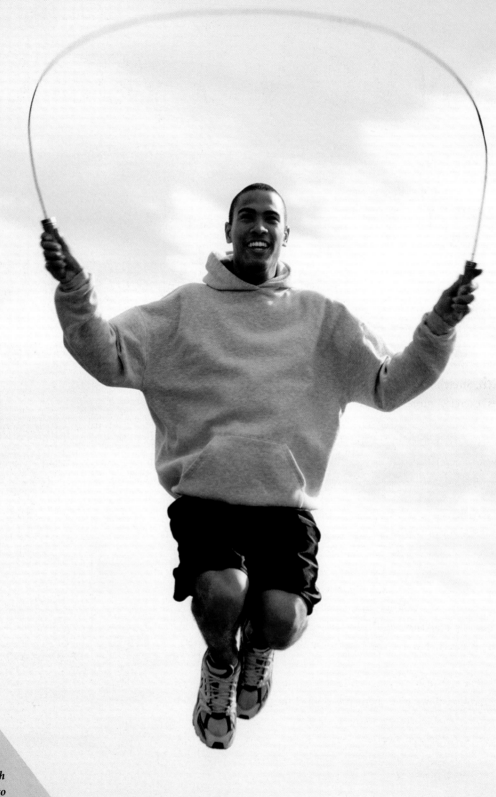

Get a jump on injury-free workouts by taking sensible precautions, such as warming up to make muscles pliant and gradually increasing intensity.

12 ways you can prevent sports injuries

STARTING UP

1. Stretch. Stretching may not directly reduce injury. But it makes exercise more tolerable and less painful by increasing your range of motion. Besides, stretching feels good. Use a slow, sustained stretch for each muscle group you're working. Hold for a count of 30. Try to stretch before the exercise and definitely after.

2. Warm up, cool down. Warm muscles are more pliant and less prone to tear. Five minutes of warm-up at a fairly easy intensity should be adequate. Do a little more in the morning or on cold days. After a workout, walk or continue your activity at a low intensity until your heart rate drops to 10 to 15 beats per minute above your resting rate. Never stop exercising suddenly—doing so can trigger a potentially dangerous drop in your blood pressure.

3. Progress gradually. "Our bodies really are remarkable at adapting if we give them the opportunity," says Russell Pate, Ph.D., past president of the American College of Sports Medicine. "But when we impose too much activity and physical stress too soon, we can easily exceed our capacity to adapt." To progress safely, increase workout duration, intensity, or distance by no more than 10 percent per week; if you've taken a break from exercising, restart at 50 to 75 percent of your previous level.

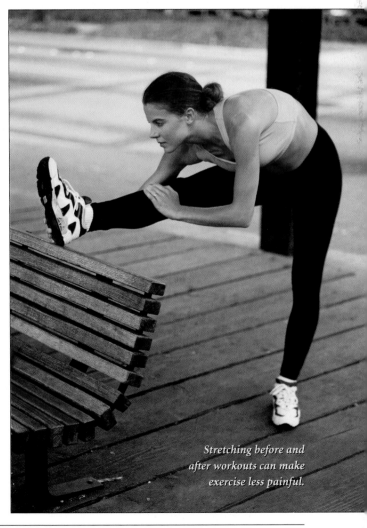

Stretching before and after workouts can make exercise less painful.

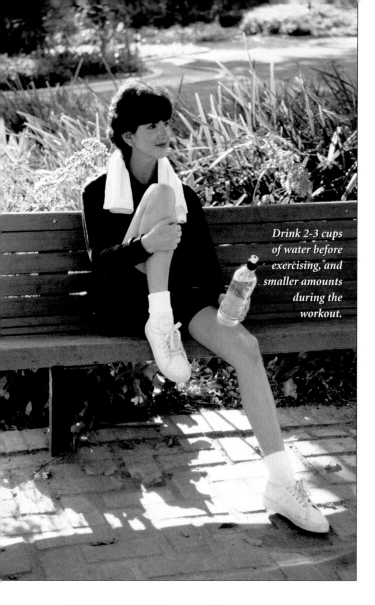

Drink 2-3 cups of water before exercising, and smaller amounts during the workout.

6. …But not too hydrated. If you drink too much water or other low-sodium drinks during a long-duration activity such as a marathon or a grueling set of singles tennis, you can put yourself at risk for hyponatremia (low blood sodium), a potentially life-threatening condition. When you're sweating profusely, it's important to replace not only fluids but also the electrolytes sodium and chloride. Try tomato juice or sports drinks, which contain sodium.

7. Stand and breathe properly. Stand up straight for weight-bearing activities like treadmill walking, elliptical training, and aerobics. Leaning forward puts undue strain on the lower back. For strength training, keep the neck relaxed and head turned frontward. Avoid locking your joints or bending them more than 90 degrees during squats, leg presses, and dips. Avoid moving parts of the body that aren't being exercised, especially the back. For weight lifting, abdominal exercises, and other strength training, exhale when you exert yourself and inhale when returning to the original relaxed position. Never hold your breath; that can drive up your blood pressure.

8. Avoid excessive reps. Unless you're a bodybuilder or serious athlete, doing one set of a strength exercise twice a week may be all you need. Extra sets increase the risk of injury and provide little added benefit. The American College of Sports Medicine defines a set as 8 to 12 repetitions at a resistance level that's challenging but lets you complete the set. If you're frail or over 65, substitute 10 to 15 reps at a slightly lower resistance.

GET THE RIGHT GEAR
9. Buy good shoes. Choose footwear designed for the activity you're doing—running shoes for running, tennis shoes for tennis—as well as specific brands and styles suited to your feet and gait. Older, overweight, or tender-footed people may need extra cushioning; a person whose

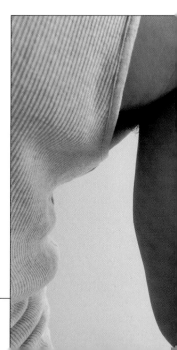

WHEN YOU'RE IN THE ZONE
4. Use exercise as prevention. "You have to train to train," Pate says. That means using exercise to prepare your body for a new or harder activity, or a return to a sport you haven't done in a while. Get ready for a ski trip with, say, jogging, weight training, and stretching.

5. Stay hydrated… Drinking plenty of liquids—especially in hot, humid weather—will prevent cramps, weakness, and dehydration. Sports-medicine experts recommend 2 to 3 cups two to three hours before you exercise and smaller amounts during the workout. Also plan to weigh yourself before and after vigorous activity to gauge fluid loss. Replace any weight you've lost with an equal amount of liquid, plus half.

feet roll inward should look for a shoe with a firm sole and back, while one whose feet roll outward may need extra cushioning or padding.

10. Wear a helmet when biking or skating.
It should sit flat across your head, with the front edge about an inch above the eyebrows. A properly adjusted helmet should stay in place when pushed upward from the front.

MONITOR CONDITIONS
11. Avoid pollution.
Exercising in air polluted with carbon monoxide, smoke, or other particles increases the risk of heart attack and stroke. Move workouts indoors on hazy, polluted days, particularly if you're being treated for cardiovascular disease. When you do exercise outside, avoid busy roads and other exhaust-heavy settings. To assess conditions in your area, check The Weather Channel's local air-quality forecast at *www.weather.com/activities/health/airquality.*

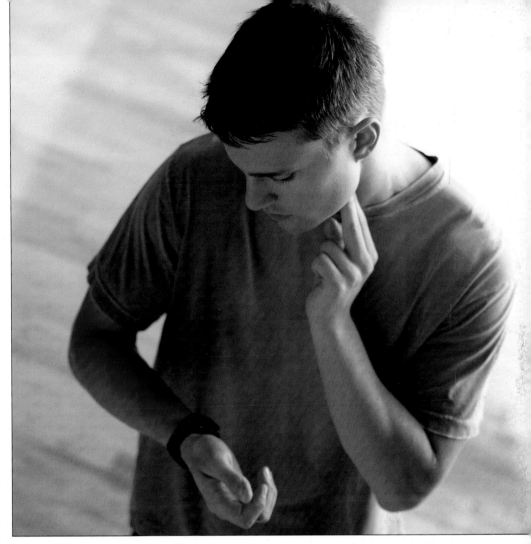

Cool down after a vigorous workout so that your heart rate drops to 10 to 15 beats per minute above your resting rate.

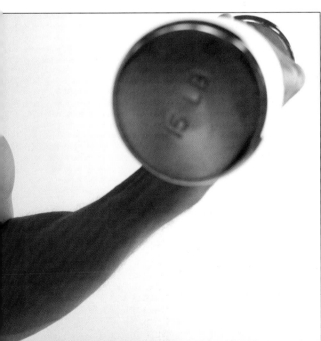

12. Let old injuries heal.
Old injuries increase the risk of a new injury to the same muscle or joint. After a sprain, wait for pain and swelling to subside. Then use daily exercises and stretches, following your doctor's advice, to rehabilitate the joint. Sports-medicine experts we consulted advise wearing a brace when you exercise for six months to reduce the risk of reinjury. Opt for a splint, available at sporting-goods stores or online. A plain elastic bandage from the pharmacy generally won't provide adequate support, and taping a joint is a job for a pro.

Don't overdo strength exercises. Doing one set of 8 to 12 repetitions, at a challenging level, twice a week may be all you need.

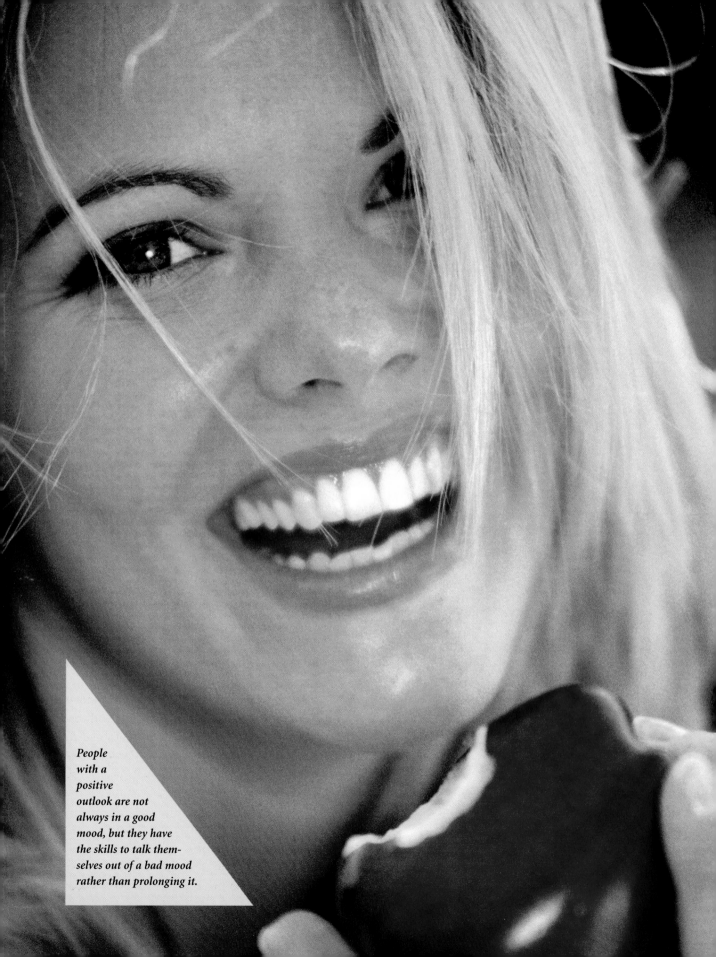

People with a positive outlook are not always in a good mood, but they have the skills to talk themselves out of a bad mood rather than prolonging it.

Happier and healthier?

Your physical well-being may reflect your mental outlook.

Happier people are often healthier people, and not just because their good health improves their mood. A growing body of observational research suggests that people who are more optimistic, less hostile, and more satisfied in youth are less likely to develop chronic diseases decades later. Similar studies also suggest that in later stages of adulthood, mental states can influence health events ranging from the minor to the life threatening.

None of this research would be particularly useful if mental outlook were a fixed quality that individuals could not improve or modify. Enter the "positive psychology" movement, which contends that people can learn optimism and happiness at any age. Until fairly recently, psychological study tended to focus solely on mental disorders, such as depression and anxiety, at the expense of inquiry into whether people without disorders could improve the positive mental states, such as happiness, strength, and hope, that make life worth living. Recent work in positive psychology has investigated the factors that distinguish happy from less

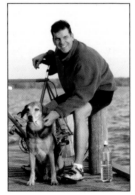

Research shows that owning a pet may help keep stress levels down.

happy people. Those insights can be helpful for people who want to boost their joy factor, though there isn't much evidence yet about which methods work best long term.

Grounded in scientific research, positive psychology should be distinguished from the kind of mind-over-matter thinking that promised that mental affirmations could cure cancer or warned that people "can't afford the luxury of a negative thought." People with a positive mental outlook are not in a good mood all of the time. But they do have the skills to talk themselves out of a bad mood rather than prolonging it, to take a self-affirming view of both negative and positive events, and to become absorbed in challenging activities. Clinical experience suggests there are practical methods you can use to brighten your mental outlook.

OPTIMISM PAYS OFF

Dozens of studies have correlated a positive mental outlook with various health outcomes. For example, there's evidence that people who are happier or more optimistic:

Pessimistic vs. optimistic interpretations of life events

How you interpret positive and negative life events is the crux of your mental outlook. If you make a mistake, do you call yourself "stupid" or say you're off your game? If you succeed at a project, is it an accident or a reflection of your inner talent? Becoming aware of your "self-talk" tendencies can help you train yourself to think more optimistically. "People who master this technique are two to eight times less likely to become depressed when they encounter setbacks," says Martin Seligman, Ph.D., professor of psychology at the University of Pennsylvania. The examples below are adapted from Seligman's book *Authentic Happiness* (Free Press, 2002).

Is it temporary or permanent?
Optimists see negative events as temporary, and positive ones as permanent.

	Pessimistic	Optimistic
Despite trying to stick to a diet, you gain weight over the holidays, and you can't lose it.	Diets don't work.	The diet I tried didn't work.
You win a tennis match.	My opponent got tired.	I'm a good player.

Is it specific or pervasive?
Optimists see negative events as specific, and positive ones as pervasive.

	Pessimistic	Optimistic
You miss an important engagement.	Sometimes my memory fails me.	I sometimes forget to check my appointment book.
You run for a community office position and win.	I devoted a lot of time and energy to campaigning.	I work hard at everything I do.

Is it hopeless or hopeful?
Hopeful people view negative events as temporary and specific, positive events as permanent and pervasive.

	Pessimistic	Optimistic
You and your spouse get into an argument.	He/she is a tyrant.	He/she was in a bad mood.
You get a promotion at work.	I'm lucky.	I'm talented.

• **Have stronger immunity.** Researchers in 2003 assessed the emotional styles of 334 healthy volunteers, then administered a squirt of rhinovirus (a germ that

Optimists tend to have stronger immunity, are less likely to die of chronic disease, and live longer.

causes colds) in the nose of each participant. Those who scored high on measures of energy, happiness, and relaxation were significantly less likely to develop colds, regardless of their health practices.

• **Are less likely to die of chronic disease.** A decade-long study of some 400 men with HIV found that those who scored highest on a scale that measured positive feelings were less likely to die at any point during the study—regardless of the extent of their illness or use of antiretroviral drugs. A few studies have yielded similar findings for cancer patients.

• **Live longer.** In a landmark study released in 2000, scientists at the Mayo Clinic analyzed the records of 839 patients who had been given psychological tests 30 years earlier. Those who scored highest on a scale of pessimism were roughly 20 percent more likely to die prematurely than were optimists. In a 2001 study, older adults who were hopeful about the future had a significantly lower death rate (11 percent) over the seven-year study period than those who said they weren't hopeful (29 percent), even after researchers adjusted for age, smoking, and health status.

STRESSED AND SICKER

On the flip side, people who are depressed, stressed, angry, or distressed tend to fare poorer. In addition to having an increased risk of heart disease (see next section), they:

• **Get sick—or feel sick—more often.** Data from one long-running, 30-year study show that, compared with optimistic people, pessimists have a higher risk of physical and mental problems.

• **Have more dental problems.** A 2003 Harvard University analysis of more than 42,000 men in the Health Professionals Follow-Up Study found that those who scored highest on an anger questionnaire were 72 percent more likely to develop periodontitis (gum disease) than those who scored lowest.

• **Heal slower from surgery.** A small New Zealand study in the journal *Psychosomatic Medicine* found that patients who were worried before undergoing hernia surgery reported slower, more painful recoveries than those who were less worried. The stressed patients also scored significantly lower on an objective marker of recovery: the levels of the repair protein interleukin-1 in their wound fluid.

• **Are more likely to get Alzheimer's disease.** In a December 2003 study in the journal *Neurology*, involving nearly 800 older people, those most prone to psychological distress—including anxiety, anger, depression, and feelings of helplessness—were twice as likely to develop Alzheimer's as those who were least prone to such feelings.

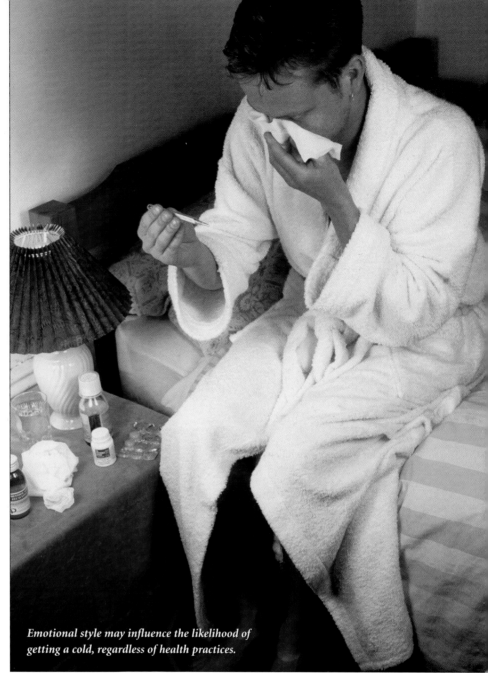

Emotional style may influence the likelihood of getting a cold, regardless of health practices.

HOW FEELINGS AFFECT PHYSIOLOGY

The mechanism through which troubled psychological states can influence health is clearest within the cardiovascular system. Substantial research has tied hostility, anger, impatience, and stress to increased heart risk; somewhat lesser evidence suggests that depression and social isolation may also harm the heart.

High levels of emotional stress, particularly anger, cause a surge in certain hormones, such as adrenaline and cortisol, that prepare your body to face an emergency. That surge causes physiological changes that can, in turn, trigger a heart attack or stroke, especially in people whose arteries are already clogged. Mental duress may also contribute to the development of disease by encouraging unhealthy lifestyle choices that increase heart risk—such as drinking, smoking, overeating, and not exercising.

Negative emotions may begin to affect risk factors as early as one's teens. In a study of more than 3,300 people published in the *Journal of the American Medical Association*, hostile and impatient young adults were nearly twice as likely as their mellower peers to develop hypertension over a 15-year period.

WHAT CAN YOU FIX?

Thus far there has been little research into whether individuals can change their mental outlook and, if so, whether this improves their health. In the book *Authentic Happiness* (Free Press, 2002), University of Pennsylvania psychology professor Martin Seligman, Ph.D., argues that our

As long as basic needs are met, studies show wealth has surprisingly little effect on happiness.

overall level of happiness depends on three factors: inborn tendencies, circumstances, and factors under our control.

Research suggests that we're born with a hardwired emotional profile, or "happiness thermostat." This is a base state of happiness, a "fixed and largely inherited level to which we invariably revert," writes Seligman. The base state may persist despite strokes of fortune or misfortune. For example, one study shows that over time, winners of large lottery prizes are no happier than non-winners. And people paralyzed after spinal-cord injuries wind up only slightly less happy, on average, than individuals who aren't so affected, according to Seligman. One's personal happiness range also appears largely independent of material wealth or other "comfortable life" factors. As long as a person's basic economic needs are met, money has surprisingly little effect on happiness.

Life events can trigger or protect against certain inborn tendencies, such as a tendency toward depression or anxiety. And some circumstances—such as extreme poverty, the death of a child, or caring for a relative with Alzheimer's disease—do have a long-range depressing effect on happiness levels.

While it may not be possible to modify your genetic inheritance or control your external circumstances, it may be possible to modify your mental outlook and response to life events. For example, clinical trials have tested the ability of meditation and other behavioral interventions to reduce hostility in heart patients; they've found that these techniques not only reduce measures of hostility but also may lower blood pressure and possibly reduce the risk of heart-attack recurrence.

Here are some of the ways psychologists believe that you can increase your happiness quotient, and perhaps simultaneously improve your health.

Cultivating positive emotion. Both your thinking and your activities affect your mental state. Thought patterns may be more amenable to change and control than many of us realize.

Meditation is a good relaxation method for coping with stress.

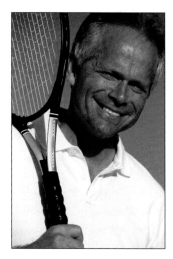

People who exercise regularly are better equipped to handle everyday ups and downs.

Just as you can interrupt an overtalkative friend, you may be able to interrupt your own negative thoughts and interpretations of the world and substitute more positive ones, using what psychologists call "self-talk." Gaining a measure of control may take persistence and perhaps professional counseling, but the mood improvement may be substantial.

• **Rewrite your past.** Research has shown that our memories seem to be mood-related. In other words, when you're in a bad mood, it's easy to remember all your other problems and grievances against the world, while when you're in a good mood, it's easy to recall other good times. So a conscious effort to dwell on good recent and long-term memories may have a powerful effect on your daily mood. Such simple measures as cultivating a sense of gratitude by "counting your blessings" each day may help amplify positive memories. So may efforts to celebrate small victories and achievements—even something as simple as patting yourself on the back. And forgiving and forgetting unpleasant experiences may help mute those memories.

• **Project a brighter future.** What do you say to yourself when you misplace your keys? If what springs to mind is "I'm an idiot," then you're interpreting the bad event as something permanent and universal, a pessimistic view likely to decrease your happiness. The remedy is to argue yourself into a more optimistic explanation: "I'm not stupid. There are many things I do well. I'm just tired and stressed today."

When it comes to responding to positive events, however, the opposite approach is best. If, for example, you've gotten a compliment or a promotion at work, it's OK to generalize. Instead of thinking "I'm just lucky" or "That last report must have impressed the boss," tell yourself, "This is a reward for all my talent, leadership ability, and hard work."

Finding "flow" in free time

The table below shows the percentage of time that each leisure activity resulted in a "flow" state, a peak experience of satisfaction that occurs when challenge and skill levels are both high. Results are from a study of 824 U.S. teenagers responding at 27,000 moments; participants were paged on beepers at random times through the day and asked to record what they were doing and feeling.

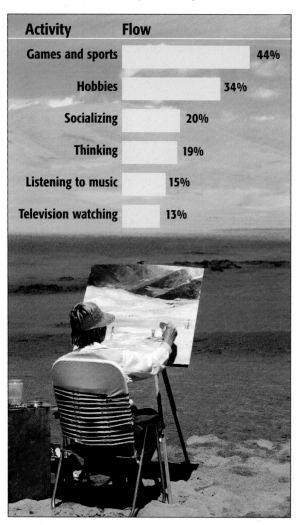

Activity	Flow
Games and sports	44%
Hobbies	34%
Socializing	20%
Thinking	19%
Listening to music	15%
Television watching	13%

• **Improve the present**. Making room in your day for more genuinely rewarding activities is another important tactic. A lasting source of happiness comes from entering a state of "flow," in which you're so absorbed in an activity that you lose your self-consciousness and even awareness of time. That occurs most readily when you're actively engaged, either mentally or physically, in activities that use favorite skills and are challenging enough to ward off boredom, but not so difficult that you become anxious.

Research amassed over the past two decades by Mihaly Csikszentmihalyi, Ph.D.—who coined the "flow" concept and currently serves as a professor of psychology at Claremont Graduate University—and his colleagues shows that activities that foster lasting happiness tend to involve creativity, exploration, imagination, strategy, and discovery.

Too often people "get trapped in life doing things that we think we have to do even if we don't like them," says Csikszentmihalyi. "We give up the things we enjoy and end up with a very thin life." To change that, you need to seek out fulfilling activities. Consider one you really enjoyed doing years ago, perhaps painting, reading, gardening, or traveling, but gave up as the pressures of adult life took over. Also think about something you've never had a chance to do, such as learning another language, going on an archaeological dig, or starting an antique-car rehabilitation service in your garage, suggests Csikszentmihalyi. Sample a range of activities you never considered before, consulting the local paper or a nearby community center for ideas. Sign up for a day trip to a nearby ghost town or state park; join a hiking club; tour your city's architectural landmarks. Or volunteer to teach others something you

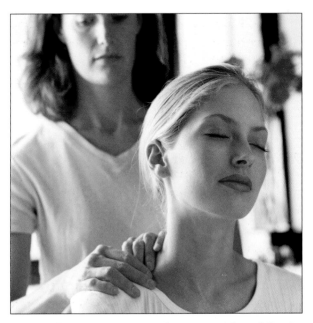

Try a soothing massage as part of your personal portfolio of strategies for coping with anger.

already know: That, Csikszentmihalyi says, may bring the best fulfillment there is.

Managing negative experiences.
Along with increasing positive thinking and activities, it's important to have tactics for dealing with the stresses of modern life. The way you manage your response to stressful events can either strain or help protect your health.

Anger and hostility are among the most dangerous responses to stress because they strain the cardiovascular system and can prompt reckless and destructive behavior. Taming those emotions involves reasoning with yourself and determining whether your rage is called for and, if so, how to deal with it constructively. Redford Williams, M.D., director of the Behavioral Medicine Research Center at Duke University, recommends asking yourself the following questions when someone does something that makes you angry:

1. **Is this important?**
2. **Is anger appropriate in this situation?**
3. **Is there anything I can do to modify the situation?**
4. **Would it be worthwhile to have a confrontation?**

If you answered yes to all four questions, you need to practice assertion: Find a constructive way to ask the offending person to change his or her behavior, whether it's a friend who just insulted you, a store clerk who says you can't return an item, or a spouse who tells you to run an errand when you're exhausted. Stay calm and rational as you make a specific request for the outcome you desire.

However, if you answered no to any of the four questions, it may pay to avoid a confrontation and use techniques to quiet your emotions. Talking to yourself ("Hey, this isn't that important!"), exercising, breathing deeply, consciously relaxing your muscles, and seeking support by talking to a friend are some options.

Acting out your feelings for the sake of catharsis is not recommended. "Punching a bag, yelling and screaming, hitting something—these types of things do nothing but make you more likely to behave aggressively afterward," Williams says. In one study, subjects who were verbally insulted and then opted to vent their anger on a punching bag acted more aggressively later than those who declined to punch.

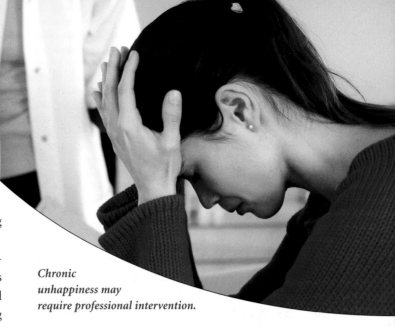

Chronic unhappiness may require professional intervention.

While a variety of techniques have the proven potential to help people cope with stress, more studies are needed to determine which techniques work best, for whom, and for how long. To put together your own portfolio of coping strategies, consider drawing from the following areas:

- **Meditation, relaxation training, yoga, tai-chi.** These all involve "mindfulness," the art of concentrating on the present moment and tuning out external factors.

- **Cognitive training.** A therapist or an adult education course may be able to help you learn to thwart a stress reaction (pounding heart, quick breathing, increased blood pressure) by reasoning with yourself and changing your thought processes. One commonly recommended cognitive tool is "thought stopping," in which you interrupt your worry or anger by literally telling yourself to stop, either aloud or under your breath.

- **Social support.** Club membership, religious or civic activities, volunteer work, or just a few close friends can help protect you from the effects of stress on the body. Animal support counts too: Researchers at the State University of New York at Buffalo found that overall, people with a pet had lower stress levels than those who did not own a pet.

- **Exercise.** People who get regular aerobic exercise have lower levels of stress hormones and smaller increases in heart rate and blood pressure under mental duress. Exercise works as a long-term antidote as well as a quick stress fix.

- **Treatment options.** Chronic anger, hostility, and unhappiness may reflect a serious underlying problem, such as depression or an anxiety disorder. In those cases, individual or group therapy and/or drug therapy may be indicated.

SUMMING UP

There is much observational evidence linking mental outlook to health outcomes. At this point, however, most strategies for improving mental outlook are based only on clinical experience. It's not yet clear whether it's possible for most people to improve their happiness levels, and, more important, if doing so can have a positive impact on their health.

There is, however, fairly good evidence that frequent hostility and anger can stress the cardiovascular system. Learning to cope better with stress has been shown to help lower blood pressure and decrease the risk of heart disease.

People interested in measures to boost their mental outlook should consider the following:

- Cultivate positive feelings by focusing on good memories rather than bad, seeking activities that provide engaging experiences, and learning to use an optimistic explanatory style.

- Create personal strategies for coping with stress, such as mindfulness practices (e.g. meditation), cognitive techniques, social support, and exercise.

- Seek professional help if your negative emotions and outlook seriously interfere with functioning or life satisfaction.

RESOURCES

- A range of free self-tests to assess optimism, happiness, and other positive emotions are available on *www.authentichappiness.org*, the companion Web site to Martin Seligman's book. You'll need to provide an e-mail address and demographic information to register. Results are confidential.

- The Web site *www.williamslifeskills.com* provides an overview of programs, workshops, and other resources to help people build strong relationships and overcome anger and other negative emotions.

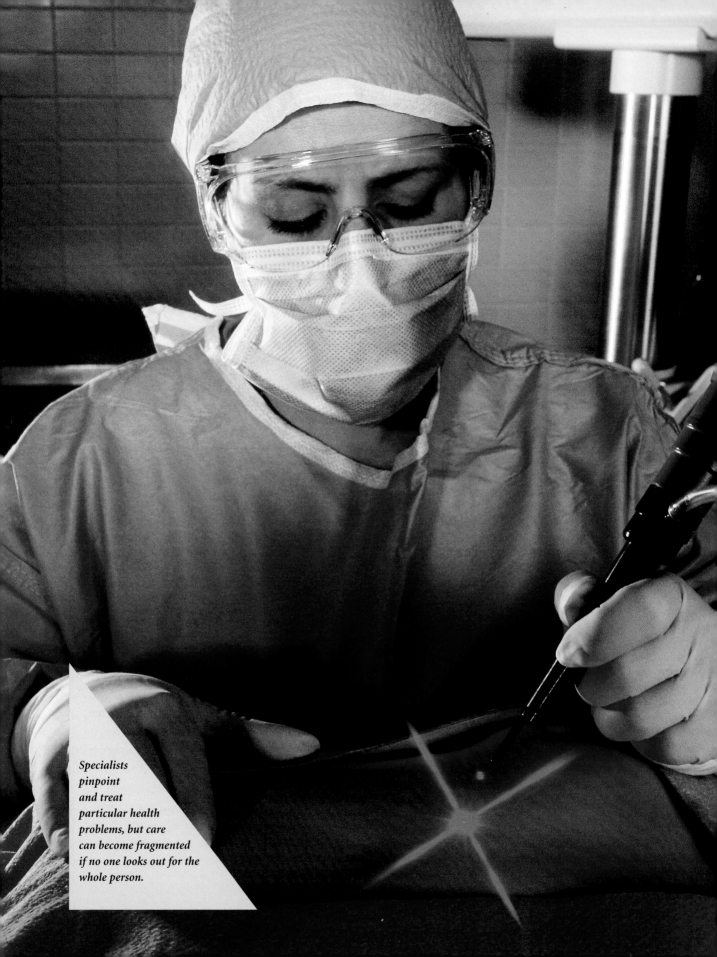

Specialists pinpoint and treat particular health problems, but care can become fragmented if no one looks out for the whole person.

When do you need a specialist?

How to get the most from your health-care team—including your regular doctors.

Throughout the past decade or two, patients seeking care from a medical specialist often ran into a formidable roadblock: their primary-care physician, pressured by insurers to cut costs by restricting access to experts. "Dr. Welby had turned into Dr. No," says Alice Gosfield, a prominent health-insurance analyst. Recently, though, that constraint has eased considerably, in part because angry patients, politicians, and providers rebelled.

Patients should indeed seek specialists in many cases: Research suggests that those physicians tend to follow treatment guidelines more closely than generalists do and, partly as a result, provide superior care for many health problems.

But specialist care has important shortcomings. Specialists tend to recommend more tests and treatments, including a greater number of needless ones, so they may

Specialists' deeper and more-current knowledge can translate into better patient outcomes.

waste patients' time and cause them more anxiety, as well as increase costs to insurers. In addition, getting care from multiple specialists can create a fragmented approach in which no one is caring for the whole person. That can be both emotionally disturbing and medically inappropriate, as problems are overlooked, duplicate tests are ordered, and incompatible medications are prescribed.

This report will help you determine when you need a specialist and how to find the best available practitioner. And we'll describe how to forge generalists and specialists into a collaborative team that maximizes the best from each one.

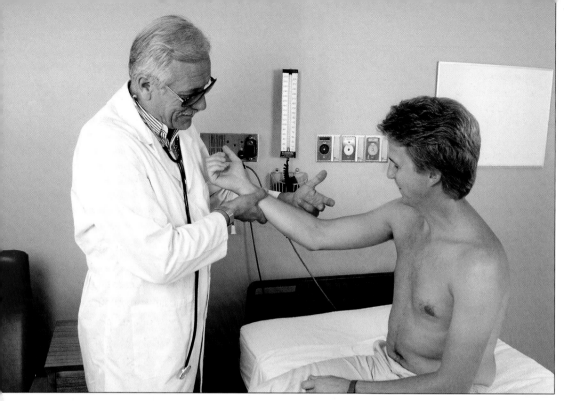

Start with your primary-care physician, who can help determine whether or not you need a specialist.

WHEN A GENERALIST SUFFICES

Your primary-care doctor—usually a family practice physician or general internist—may have enough experience and training to adequately treat many conditions. Indeed, the numerous evidence-based practice guidelines written in the past few years make it increasingly feasible for generalists to manage even some serious and complex problems—provided they take the time to read and follow those guidelines. Moreover, generalists routinely handle a number of problems at least as competently as specialists do.

For example, most people who have lower back pain or osteoarthritis of the knee fare no better when cared for by an orthopedist. Heartburn patients in one study did just as well with a nurse's advice as with a gastroenterologist's. And generalists are obviously the best choice for colds, the flu, sprains, and other everyday problems.

THE SPECIALISTS' EDGE

It's clearly wise to see a specialist when you have a health problem that most general-practice doctors see only occasionally. For example, people with lupus or multiple sclerosis are probably better off seeing a rheumatologist or

neurologist, respectively, at least periodically. (For information about particularly rare diseases, contact the National Organization of Rare Disorders at 203-744-0100 or *www.rarediseases.org*.)

Even with some of the more common conditions, the medical literature has become so huge, and medical technology so complex, that it's often hard for generalists to keep up. Indeed, considerable research suggests that specialists provide care that is more consistent with recently published research and guidelines for a number of common problems—including asthma, diabetes, psoriasis, stomach ulcers, and several forms of

If you have a disease unfamiliar to most generalists, such as lupus or multiple sclerosis, it's wise to see a specialist.

heart disease and cancer. In addition, the advanced training and extensive experience of specialists helps them recognize subtleties that a generalist might miss.

That deeper and more-current knowledge can translate into better patient outcomes. For example, a study of some 39,000 patients who had suffered an ischemic stroke (caused by a blocked artery) found that those treated by a neurologist were about one-third less likely to die within 90 days than those treated by a generalist. And among nearly 2,000 adults with asthma, patients seen mainly by an allergist reported substantially fewer hospitalizations and visits to the emergency room.

Controlling patient visits to specialists

During the 1980s, specialist care increased substantially while care by family practitioners declined. But both trends leveled off in the 1990s, as insurers tried to cut costs by limiting access to specialists. (The numbers of visits to internists, pediatricians, and obstetricians was steady during the two decades, possibly because they're both generalists and specialists.) In theory, figures for the last few years, which are not yet available, may show a renewed trend toward specialization because insurers have been forced to relax their restrictions.

In general, consider consulting a specialist if:

• You have a life-threatening condition, such as cancer, or have suffered a serious event, such as a heart attack or stroke.

• You have an uncommon disease—or one that your primary-care physician has rarely treated.

• Your problem worsens or hasn't improved, despite several attempted treatments or medications.

• Diagnostic tests fail to find the cause of your symptoms.

• You research your disorder thoroughly and suspect that your current treatment is inadequate or inappropriate.

• Your doctor can't answer all of your questions about the problem.

• Your individual needs warrant special attention. For example, a professional athlete or dancer might want to see an orthopedist for a simple ankle sprain, while the average person might not; and someone planning a visit to a developing or tropical country may want to see a travel medicine specialist to make sure he or she gets the appropriate inoculations and thorough information on infectious-disease prevention.

THE POWER OF TEAMWORK

Even when you need one or more specialists, don't abandon your primary-care physician. In many cases, all that's needed is one or two visits with a specialist, who may simply suggest tests or medication and set up a maintenance plan for you and your primary doctor to follow. If ongoing visits are required, your regular physician still plays an essential role by supplementing and reviewing the specialist's care.

In some cases a generalist may be able to rein in a specialist who's recommending overaggressive treatment. Until recently, for example, gynecologists prescribed supplemental estrogen for postmenopausal women far more often than general-practice physicians, despite a lack of evidence from clinical trials supporting that practice. Similarly, orthopedists tend to order more X-rays for low-back pain, though such tests are rarely needed.

And unless your primary doctor stays involved, specialist care can become splintered, especially when you

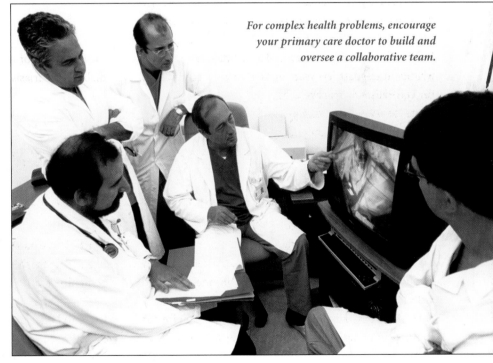

For complex health problems, encourage your primary care doctor to build and oversee a collaborative team.

have several doctors focusing on separate body parts. For example, someone who goes to a cardiologist for high blood pressure, an orthopedist for back pain, an endocrinologist for diabetes, and a neurologist for headaches may never learn that a single cause, such as a pituitary tumor,

How far are you willing to travel?

"When people learn they have a serious disease, their first reaction is often, 'Where's the best place in the world to go for this?' " says Eileen Coan, resource director for The Gathering Place, a Cleveland organization that helps recently diagnosed cancer patients. "They're often willing to travel anywhere, and they assume that's what they'll have to do," she says.

Finding a good doctor and, if necessary, a good hospital are indeed essential when you're seriously ill. But for the vast majority of illnesses, you can usually find excellent care fairly

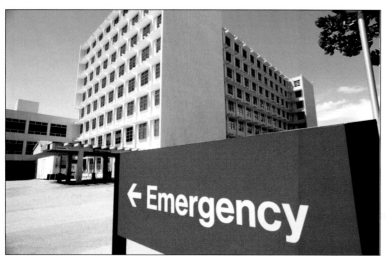

close to home, especially if you live in or near a big city.

Traveling for health care, however, may offer advantages in certain cases. For example, you might have a rare condition that's adequately treated by only a few experts worldwide. Or you've searched the medical literature and discussed your findings with local doctors, and you're convinced that a particular physician or hospital offers hope you can't get nearby. Or you're simply determined to get the very best possible care, regardless of the cost or inconvenience.

In those cases, here are the main difficulties you'll face and what it takes to overcome them.

• No or limited insurance coverage

Managed-care plans often force members to use specific hospitals and turn efforts to go elsewhere into protracted battles. If possible, consider switching to a plan that allows more choice. But check the fine print for waiting periods and exclusions of preexisting conditions. Or appeal your existing plan's restriction (see Consumers Union's free "Consumer Guide to Handling Disputes with Your Employer or Private Health Plan" online at *www.ConsumersUnion.org/health/hmo-review*).

• Travel expenses

Health insurance rarely pays for travel and lodging. However, such costs may be tax-deductible as medical expenses. The nonprofit Cancer Research Institute (800-992-2623, *www.cancerresearch.org/hbrdtran.html*) maintains a list of organizations that offer free or reduced rates for travel and lodging for such medical care. Finally, contact the hospital's social-service department, local charities, or disease-specific support groups about the availability of free or low-cost lodging.

• Isolated care

Without your primary-care doctor nearby, you're particularly susceptible to disjointed care from unfamiliar specialists. That isolation can be especially severe if friends or family can't accompany you. Ask the hospital's admissions department if there's a "hospitalist" on staff, a doctor who serves as a temporary primary-care physician. Also ask what records or paperwork you'll need, and ask your local primary physician to help you gather and send them. To ensure appropriate care when you return, involve your local doctors beforehand and ask your main specialist at the new hospital to recommend a specialist near home, if appropriate.

actually links them all—a connection that a generalist may be more likely to spot.

Similarly, a primary-care doctor who reviews the treatment provided by multiple specialists may uncover redundant tests and incompatible drug prescriptions.

That oversight is especially essential in the hospital, when you're likely to be cared for by a phalanx of unfamiliar specialists who communicate mainly through cryptic notes in your chart.

Finally, a specialist may treat individual problems well

but neglect your overall health. That's a particular problem in older people or those with a chronic disease, who often have multiple health problems. Indeed, studies of three such disorders—depression, heart failure, and rheumatoid arthritis—found that while people cared for by specialists fared better than others, those who also saw their primary-care doctor showed the best overall improvement.

To get the most from your team of health-care professionals, make sure to tell your primary-care doctor and specialists all the symptoms you have, all the drugs you take, and all procedures you've undergone. Expect your primary-care doctor to thoroughly review your care at least once a year and, if possible, whenever you're in the hospital for more than a day or so.

And for complex health problems, encourage your primary-care doctor to build and oversee a collaborative team of physician and nonphysician specialists, as appropriate. For example, people with diabetes often require an endocrinologist, an ophthalmologist, and a podiatrist to manage the disease and its complications. They also need a dietitian and diabetes-educator (usually a nurse) to assist in the needed lifestyle changes.

Similarly, individuals who experience chronic pain may need a neurologist, anesthesiologist, and psychiatrist. (For more on the non-M.D.s you may want to include in your team, see the accompanying item, "Specialists in the human touch," on page 155.)

HOW TO PICK A SPECIALIST

When you're sick or uncertain enough to need a specialist you obviously want to find the best one you can. If you're on Medicare or have free-choice insurance—or lots of money—you can generally choose any specialist you want. One way is simply to ask your doctor to recommend someone.

For complicated or unusual problems, ask your doctor for the name of an expert recognized nationwide or search the

Choose a specialist with a good reputation for technical skill and few patient complaints.

medical literature to find someone who has published major articles about your problem. Then contact that physician and ask him or her to recommend someone in your area; in some cases you might even consider traveling to consult with or be treated by the out-of-town expert (see "How far are you willing to travel?" on the facing page).

If you don't have a solid recommendation, however, it's wise to learn all you can about the prospective consultants. That may also be necessary if your insurance requires you to choose from a list of names that your doctor may not recognize.

Start out by contacting the American Board of Medical Specialties (866-275-2267 or *www.certifieddoctor.org*) to

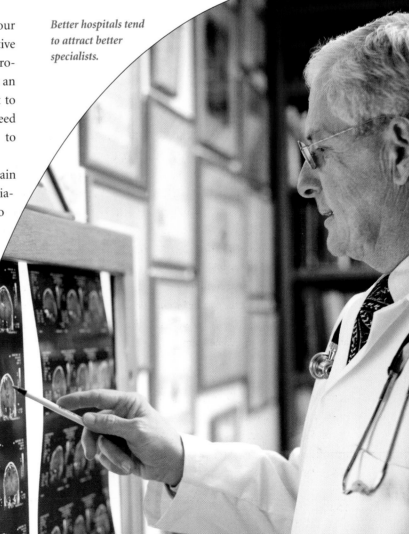

Better hospitals tend to attract better specialists.

learn whether the physician is board-certified in a particular medical specialty. Certification means the person has completed an approved residency program and passed a detailed written exam in at least one of 24 specialty areas.

The American Medical Association's "Doctor-Finder" Web site (*www.ama-assn.org/aps/amahg.htm*) can provide additional information, notably where the physician underwent residency training. Doctors trained at big-city university medical centers likely have more experience with a wider variety of cases than those trained in smaller hospitals.

Administrators in Medicine (*www.docfinder.org*), an association of state medical-board executive directors, provides state-by-state information about professional misconduct by physicians. Click on your state, then search by the doctor's name. Or follow the appropriate link to your state's medical board, and contact the agency directly.

Meanwhile, try using your own contacts or those of someone you know to get in touch with a health professional who works with the specialist. Then ask whether the physician:

- Has a history of patient complaints or malpractice suits.
- Has a good reputation for technical skill.
- Is willing to consult with other specialists and refer patients to other doctors.

Finally, talk with the specialist in person. Ask if he or she belongs to any medical-specialty societies, such as the American College of Cardiology or the American Academy of Dermatology. While requirements for joining such groups vary, membership at least suggests that the physician has some interest in keeping up with the latest research. (To confirm membership, contact the society.)

Your general doctor can supplement and review your specialist care, checking especially for overlooked health problems, redundant tests, incompatible drugs, or overly aggressive therapies.

Most important, ask how experienced he or she is with your particular problem. For surgeons, find out how many of the operations they've performed, since studies clearly show that success rates rise and complications decline with experience. Then ask your primary-care doctor to help you interpret the numbers. Also ask which hospitals the doctor admits patients to, then check the quality of that hospital, since better hospitals tend to attract better doctors.

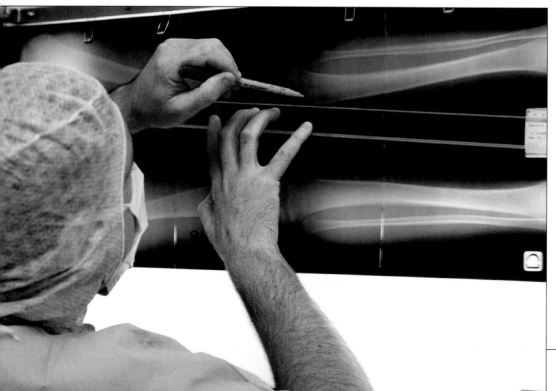

If you require surgery, ask about the specialist's experience and success rate.

Specialists in the human touch

In some cases, what you want in a health-care professional is not more expertise but more time and a more personal approach. The best choices then can be certain nonphysician health-care providers, whose main strengths lie in caring for the whole individual.

The most common of those are nurse-practitioners, certified nurse-midwives, and physician assistants. The first two are licensed registered nurses who've received additional training and, usually, graduate degrees. Most nurse-practitioners function as primary-care providers; midwives typically focus on childbirth, though some also provide general

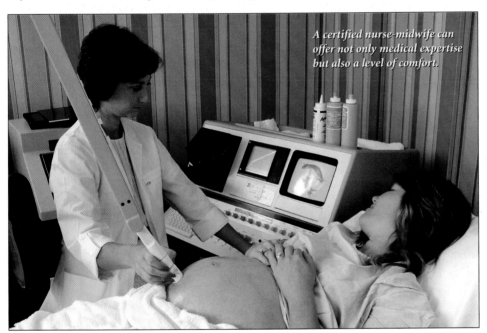

A certified nurse-midwife can offer not only medical expertise but also a level of comfort.

care to women, as gynecologists do. Both can practice independently of physicians in most states, though they must be affiliated with a doctor to whom they can refer patients when necessary. Physician assistants, who complete a two-

year postgraduate training program, work directly under a supervising physician. All three professionals can write prescriptions in all or nearly all states.

Research shows that nurse-practitioners and physician assistants are perfectly capable of evaluating and treating most commonplace medical problems, and that certified nurse-midwives safely handle low-risk pregnancies, from prenatal care through delivery. Studies have also shown that these professionals typically identify complex problems beyond their training and refer the patient to a physician.

But their main advantage is the more personal and in-depth attention each typically provides. For example, you can expect them to spend more time with you during routine visits and to supply more information on disease prevention and health maintenance. During delivery, women can expect their midwife to stay with them throughout labor. Some patients may also speak more freely and feel less intimidated than with a doctor.

To reduce the chance of inappropriate care from these professionals, it's essential that you speak up if you think your problem needs a doctor's attention—for example, if you're seriously ill, need a comprehensive checkup, or your symptoms don't improve.

SUMMING UP

Specialists often provide better care than generalists, especially for severe or uncommon conditions. But you always need a generalist, too. Your primary-care physician can treat many common problems at least as effectively as specialists do, usually at less cost. And when you need a specialist, your regular doctor can supplement and review your specialist care, checking especially for overlooked health problems, redundant tests, incompatible drugs, or overly aggressive therapies.

When seeking a specialist, check his or her reputation by contacting the sources mentioned in this report and by asking people you know, especially health-care professionals, about their experiences.

Is mold making you sick?

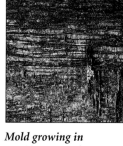

Mold growing in walls can cause respiratory problems.

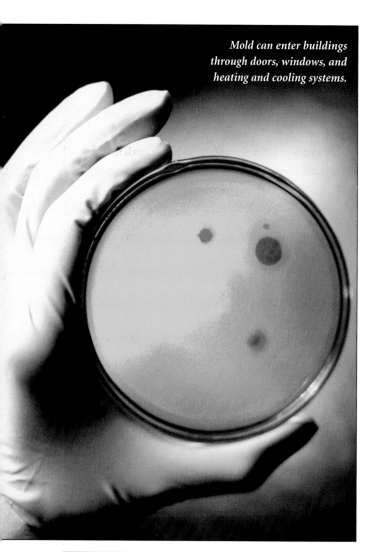

Mold can enter buildings through doors, windows, and heating and cooling systems.

Mold is big news—and big business—these days. The discovery of "toxic mold" in homes and other buildings has prompted lawsuits, school closings, and a burgeoning industry of mold consultants, mold cleaners, and mold-detection products—all based largely on claims that breathing moldy air can gravely harm your health.

While the headlines have hyped mold as the most dangerous indoor health risk since asbestos, science paints a fuzzier picture. It's true that inhaling indoor mold can cause certain health problems, mostly respiratory, in some people. But there's no convincing evidence that it causes such serious conditions as internal bleeding, memory loss, and chronic lethargy. And while some molds do produce toxins, researchers don't yet know whether inhaling those molds is any more harmful than inhaling ordinary molds.

THE FUNGUS AMONG US

Mold thrives in warm, dark, humid environments and spreads via spores, which can enter buildings through doors, windows, and heating and cooling systems. A spore need only land on a moist surface for growth to begin.

Since no one tracks mold prevalence, there's no way to know whether it's on the rise. In theory, though, the airtight building techniques introduced in the 1970s may make today's homes more hospitable to mold by trapping moisture and restricting air circulation. The switch from plaster to wood-based construction might also invite mold, which thrives on damp wood and wallboard. Basements are ideal fungal breeding grounds, dark and often damp; so the increasing popularity of finished basements may also theoretically up our mold exposure risk.

HEALTH EFFECTS OF MOLD

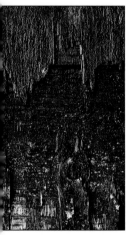

All molds can cause health problems in a minority of people. Those who are allergic to mold may experience sneezing, stuffed or runny nose, itchy eyes, or skin rash. Mold can worsen asthma or other chronic respiratory problems, and continued exposure to a damp, moldy environment can actually cause people to develop a mold allergy or asthma. Exposure to high levels of mold can irritate the eyes, skin, nose, throat, and lungs. And people with lung disease or weakened immunity may be susceptible to fungal lung infections when exposed to moldy air.

Some molds that grow indoors—such as the highly publicized Stachybotrys chartarum, sometimes called "toxic black mold"—produce mycotoxins, toxic substances that can cause illness or even death if ingested from food. Fever, headaches, fatigue, lethargy, vomiting, internal bleeding, memory loss, and other cognitive impairments have been reported in people who supposedly inhaled toxins from those molds. But experts say it's unlikely that mycotoxins in indoor environments could become airborne in high enough concentrations to produce a toxic effect. (Since all molds, toxic or not, can cause gastrointestinal problems if eaten, you should remove all visible mold from firm foods, such as hard cheese, and discard soft moldy foods, like bread.)

Several large recent reviews of the medical literature have found little or no support for claims that exposure to Stachybotrys or other toxic molds in the air causes serious or life-threatening illness. Another large review is currently underway by the Institute of Medicine for the Centers for Disease Control and Prevention.

Mold prevention and cleanup

Even if breathing in mold doesn't bother you, the damage it can do to your home, and its potential health risks for others, warrant taking the following mold-prevention steps:

- Find and fix leaks, and clean up spills and water damage within 48 hours.
- Turn on exhaust fans or open windows when showering or washing dishes.
- Keep indoor humidity below 50 percent, using air conditioners or dehumidifiers when necessary.
- Don't use wallpaper or carpets in bathrooms or other damp rooms.

If you find mold and it's not too widespread, you can probably remove it on your own, following these guidelines:

- Wear an N-95 respirator mask (available at hardware stores), rubber gloves that reach midforearm, and goggles.
- Kill mold by scrubbing hard surfaces with bleach and water (1 part bleach to 10 parts water). Dry thoroughly.
- Discard soft, porous materials that have heavy mold growth, such as wallboard, carpet, or ceiling tiles.

If you detect a strong musty or mildewy smell in your home but can't find any mold, it may be inside your walls, floors, or ceiling. Consider hiring a professional mold remover in that case. Check references and ask the professional to follow federal mold cleanup recommendations, available at *www.epa.gov/iaq/molds/mold_remediation.html*. (Don't bother having the mold tested, since there are currently no standards for "safe" or "unsafe" mold levels.)

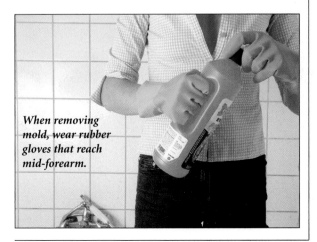

When removing mold, wear rubber gloves that reach mid-forearm.

Get more from your daily walk

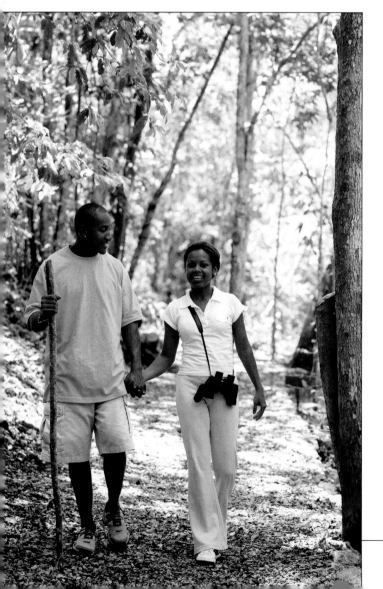

For most people, brisk walking for 30 minutes most days of the week is a convenient, pleasant way to fill your quota for aerobic exercise. The trouble is that fitness walking can become so routine that it's easy to forget you're exercising and grow bored or slip into a more leisurely pace. The simple enhancements below, done as you walk, can make your outings more engaging and challenging, and add major value in the form of extra cardiovascular work or toning for specific areas of your body.

ADD WEIGHT

Walking with some extra weight instantly boosts the aerobic benefit. Belts or vests with pockets for inserting weights are the safest method, since they distribute weight evenly over the upper body. Wearing a backpack filled with groceries or books also works well, as long as it's well balanced and fits properly.

However, strapping on ankle or wrist weights, or carrying hand weights, is not recommended. Those can increase the risk of injury to the joints, since they concentrate weight on only one part of the body, and can compromise the overall mechanics of your walk, potentially

Walking for 30 minutes most days of the week can be a pleasant way to get a regular cardiovascular workout.

slowing you down. Your best bet: Save the ankle, wrist, or hand weights for strength training, and rely on the safer weight-adding options above.

WORK MORE MUSCLES

With a little practice, you can add a significant amount of strengthening work to your walks without missing a step. The following moves can help you tone four of your body's major muscle groups. The "lunge walk" was recommended by Cedric Bryant, Ph.D., chief exercise physiologist for the American Council on Exercise; the other exercises come from Marilyn Bach, Ph.D., a Twin Cities-based personal trainer and co-author of *ShapeWalking: Six Easy Steps to Your Best Body* (Hunter House, 2002)

• **Stomach.** As you walk, contract your abdominal muscles for a count of 4 to 10, breathing normally and holding until the muscles fatigue. Release, then keep walking for 2 minutes without pulling in your stomach, and follow with another contraction. To practice locating and contracting your abdominals, stand with your back against a wall, fingers across your abdomen. Push your back into the wall and hold; you should feel the muscles contract under your fingers. When you can tighten them at will, you're ready to incorporate an abdominal contraction into your walk. Over time, you should be able to maintain the contraction for longer and longer.

• **Thighs.** Choose a route with a hill or steep flight of stairs at least 5 minutes into the walk. As you climb, squeeze the quadricep muscles in the front of your leg as it strikes the ground and pushes off, alternating legs as you go. A second option: Add a "lunge walk" to your regimen. Every few strides, sink into a gentle lunge, taking care to keep the knee directly above the foot. This move also tones the buttocks.

• **Upper arms.** Tie a resistance band around your waist, leaving an equal length of band on each side. Any time you stop moving forward—while waiting to cross the street, for example—grasp the ends of the band and bring the elbows slightly behind the body. Holding the elbows steady, extend one or both forearms back until the arm is almost straight. March in place to keep your heart rate up. Begin with one set of 10 repetitions per walk for each arm, then work up to two or three sets if desired.

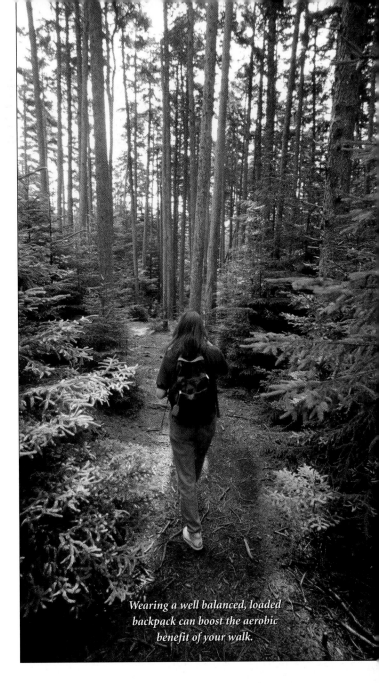

Wearing a well balanced, loaded backpack can boost the aerobic benefit of your walk.

• **Buttocks.** First try contracting your gluteal muscles while standing still, thinking of pulling each cheek forward and up. Then practice walking slowly while squeezing the gluteal muscles of the leg that's on the ground, alternating sides as you move forward. When you're ready to incorporate the contractions into your walking workout, begin with 1 minute of squeezing followed by at least 2 minutes of regular walking, gradually building up to longer contractions. Don't feel discouraged if it takes a while to get the hang of this: "It requires some concentration," Bach says.

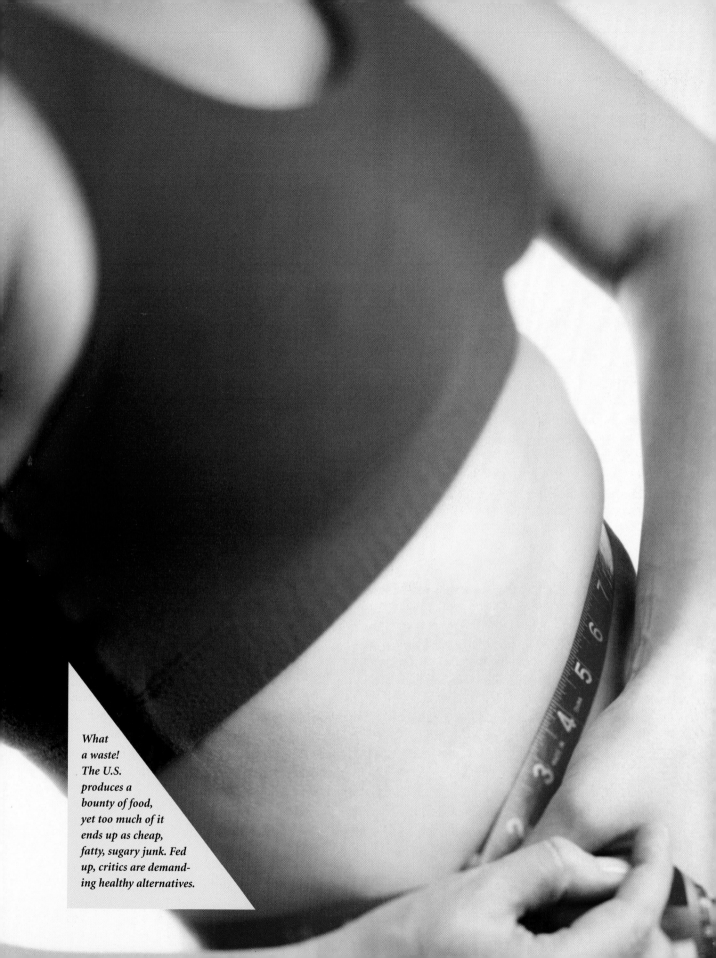

What a waste! The U.S. produces a bounty of food, yet too much of it ends up as cheap, fatty, sugary junk. Fed up, critics are demanding healthy alternatives.

Cut the Fat

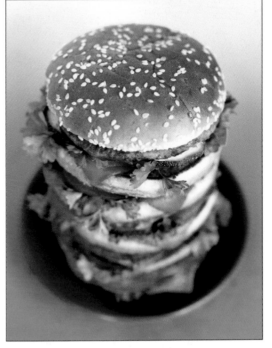

The fast-food industry stacks up as a main culprit, but it's beginning to offer some lower-fat, lower-carb meals.

It's a recipe for weight gain. Many American farms are churning out an overabundance of food, especially the foods that put on the pounds.

This bounty of corn, rice, soybeans, sugar, and wheat contribute to the availability of healthful foods at low consumer prices. But they are heavily used to create processed foods and to fatten hogs and cattle. The glut of these ingredients has enabled the food industry to market hundreds of new cheap, high-calorie snacks a year; to sell jumbo soft drinks for pennies more than smaller servings and to serve up supersized burgers, french fries, and pasta for low prices. And that, federal studies show, has distorted home cooks' sense of how much to heap on the family's dinner plates.

Cheap food translates into cheap calories, which end up growing waistlines as well as profits: 65 percent of American adults are overweight or obese, up from 47 percent 25 years ago.

Of course, no one is forcing Americans to overeat. And staying at a healthy weight takes adequate exercise as well as caloric restraint. The food and restaurant industries are heavily promoting those points in public-relations campaigns. The Grocery Manufacturers of America notes the "critical role of personal responsibility in improving fitness and nutrition." And the American Council for Fitness and Nutrition, funded by the food industry, promotes "the critical balance between fitness and nutrition." In an editorial, the newspaper *Advertising Age* said that Kentucky Fried Chicken's marketing of "breaded, fried chicken as part of a healthy diet merits special derision."

The food and restaurant industries are "letting the food part of the equation off the hook," says Kelly D. Brownell, Ph.D., chair of the department of psychology at Yale University. The ready availability and skillful marketing of cheap, tasty, high-calorie products has made it difficult, if not impossible, for many people to achieve the "balance" that food and restaurant companies so confidently prescribe.

At the very least, you need reliable nutrition information so that you can choose more healthful foods and resist the marketing messages intended to get you to overindulge. But adequate, accurate information is hard to come by:

• Food labels may disguise added sugar under confounding pseudonyms (see "Sugars hide under many names on food labels," on page 164).

• Restaurant menus don't always give you the information you need to choose meals that contain a reasonable number of calories.

• Food recommendations issued by the government may be compromised by food-industry lobbyists.

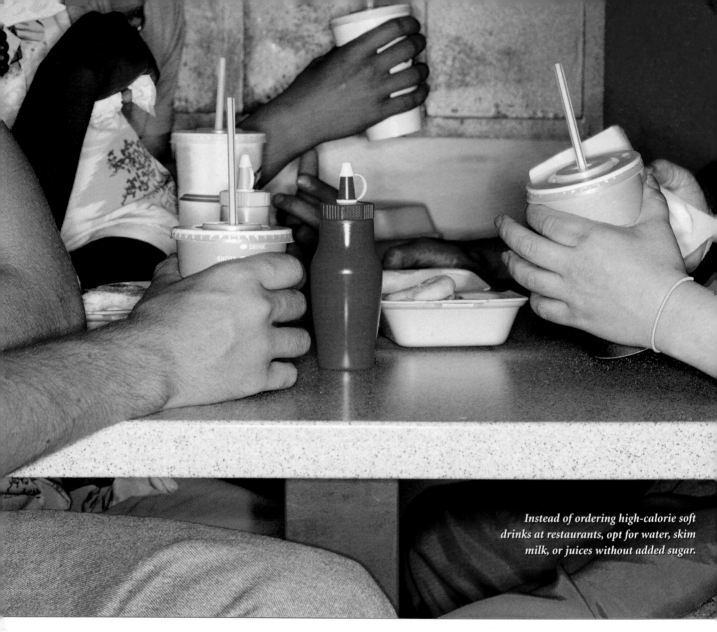

Instead of ordering high-calorie soft drinks at restaurants, opt for water, skim milk, or juices without added sugar.

Perhaps the best-kept secret is that the glut of cheap, high-calorie food is financed, in part, by your tax dollars. That's because federal farm subsidies encourage production of the very foods that we should eat less of to maintain a healthy weight.

In this environment, "the people who don't get fat are the exceptions," says Barbara Rolls, Ph.D., a professor of nutrition at Pennsylvania State University.

Portion sizes have become bloated over the last few decades.

We've uncovered and distilled what you need to know to keep the innocent act of feeding yourself and your family from becoming a threat to your health and well-being.

INDUSTRY'S HIGH-CAL HABIT

The food industry, which has prospered for years by making it cheap and easy for people to consume more calories, is on the defensive. Lawyers are filing suits against fast-food chains. Hard-hitting books, such as *Food Politics* by Marion Nestle, Ph.D., M.P.H. (University of California Press, 2002) and *Food Fight* by Brownell, the Yale professor (Contemporary Books, 2004) take the industry to task for "corporate opportunism."

Some big food companies are responding by changing the products they offer. McDonald's has introduced a successful line of entrée salads, and it is test marketing a fresh apple dip dessert and an "adult Happy Meal" that includes salad, bottled water, and a step meter to encourage more walking. Pizza Hut has added a thin crust Fit 'N Delicious pie with half the cheese. Taco Bell customers can now replace cheese with low-calorie, fat free Fiesta Salsa.

Even a critic like Brownell regards those steps as evidence that some food companies "are genuinely interested in discussion and want to make forward movement." But it may be hard for companies to kick the high-cal habit. Frito-Lay said it's developing "a wide variety of better-for-you snacks." But in 2002 it also introduced Go Snacks—Doritos, Fritos, and Cheetos packaged in reclosable plastic containers that "fit perfectly into a car's cup holder" so people can "stay on the go without going hungry."

As part of its anti-obesity initiative, Kraft Foods promised to look for ways to cut fat and calories and to take a hard look at portion sizes. But in September 2003, the company introduced supersized Easy Mac Big Pacs, "which boast 50 percent more of the delicious macaroni and cheese that teens already love."

FIGHTING PORTION DISTORTION

Bloated portions have become the norm throughout the food system, distorting our sense of the "right" amount to eat at a sitting. Judith Stern, Sc.D., a professor of nutrition at the University of California at Davis, recently compared the latest edition of *Joy of Cooking* with the 1960s-vintage edition she got as a newlywed. She was amazed to find that recipes once labeled as serving six now are labeled as serving only four. Even so, home-cooked meals are not the major source of the overeating problem. Federal studies find that people eat more calories away from home than when they eat in.

Not only are restaurant meals

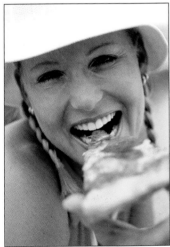

Pizza can be just as tasty if made with thinner crust and less cheese.

Overweight by the numbers

Calorie production is up

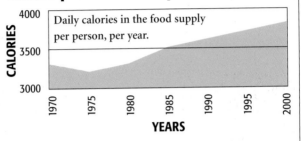

Source: USDA, Economic Research Service.

Sweetener production is up

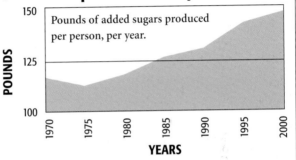

Source: USDA, Economic Research Service.

Obesity is way up

The percent of Americans who are overweight has risen slightly, but the percent who are obese has soared.

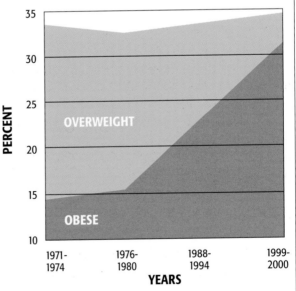

Source: HHS, National Center for Health Statistics

Sugars hide under many names on food labels

Sugars are an intrinsic part of many foods. Milk, for example, contains lactose, and fruits contain fructose. Then there are the sweeteners added to foods, either at the table, with the spoonful of sugar stirred into your coffee, or during food processing, when high-fructose corn syrup is added to foods as obvious as soft drinks and as unexpected as canned ravioli.

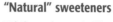

Despite heavy protest from the sugar lobby last year, the World Health Organization recommended that in a healthful diet no more than 10 percent of calories should come from sugars that aren't inherently part of a food. That works out to about 50 grams, or 13 teaspoons, as part of a 2,000-calorie-a-day diet. The average American eats more than twice that much sugar. And our consumption of added caloric sweeteners has risen 24 percent in the last 20 years.

If you want to cut back on added sugar, you'll get little help from the current U.S.-government-mandated food label. The "sugars" specified on the label include both the intrinsic and added kinds. An example: Yoplait's Yumsters strawberry low-fat yogurt is labeled as "perfect for toddlers." But each 4-ounce container includes 18 grams of sugar, compared with just 8 grams—all from milk—in the same amount of plain low-fat yogurt. The sweetened yogurt contains not only sugar, listed second on the list of ingredients, but also high-fructose corn syrup, listed fourth.

"Natural" sweeteners

While you're probably aware you should limit foods with added sugar, you may not realize just how much you're getting from juices that are labeled "all fruit" or "no added sugars." Concentrated apple or grape juice are potent sweeteners that provide just as many calories as other forms of sugar.

A cup of Mott's 100-percent apple juice contains more calories, virtually all from sugar, than the same amount of Sprite. Check calorie counts when choosing products, and keep in mind that foods and beverages labeled "all natural" may be heavily sweetened with added fruit-juice concentrates.

While fruit juices may also contain some vitamins and minerals, either naturally or through fortification, they have a lot of calories per serving and are missing many of the nutritional ingredients of whole fruit. The American Academy of Pediatrics advises that giving babies bottles filled with juice and allowing toddlers to sip from a juice box or cup for hours on end is an invitation to tooth decay and weight gain.

Adults and older children should eat whole fruit rather than juice. A cup of Mott's apple juice provides 120 calories, 28 grams of sugar, some potassium, and a small amount of vitamin C from fortification. A medium apple contains only 72 calories and half the grams of sugar (14), as well as ingredients entirely missing from the juice, such as 3 grams of fiber and the nutrients vitamin A, lutein, and beta-carotene.

more fattening, we're eating more of them than we used to. In 1977, 37 percent of the total U.S. food budget was spent on meals away from home. That figure rose to 46 percent in 2002.

The consequences are predictable:

• A long-term University of Minnesota study of 891 women, published in the October 2000 *International Journal of Obesity*, found that those who ate more frequently at fast-food restaurants consumed more calories and gained more weight than those who ate less frequently at such restaurants.

• A not-yet-published 15-year study from Harvard Medical School of more than 3,700 young adults from across the country found that eating fast food more than twice a week increased the risk of obesity by about 50 percent for whites (though not, surprisingly, for blacks).

Over the past several decades, the restaurant and snack-food industries discovered that they could attract more customers and increase profits by charging just a little bit more for a substantially larger helping. Supersizing is profitable because farm subsidies and agricultural technology have made American food the cheapest in the world in relation to our incomes. Only about 20 percent of restaurant costs are spent on food; labor and overhead costs stay the same regardless of portion size.

So portion sizes have grown. "In the mid-1950s, McDonald's offered only one size of french fries; that size is now considered "Small," and "is one-third the weight of the largest size available in 2001," wrote Lisa R. Young, Ph.D., a New York University nutritionist, in the February

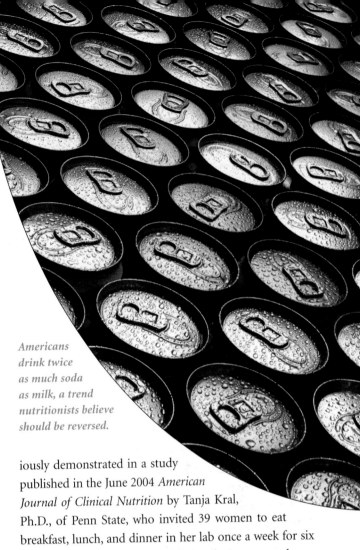

Americans drink twice as much soda as milk, a trend nutritionists believe should be reversed.

Minimize, don't supersize. Or take half the serving home to eat tomorrow.

2002 *American Journal of Public Health.* "Today's 'Large' weighs the same as the 1998 'Supersize,' and the 2001 'Supersize' weighs nearly an ounce more."

Some restaurant portions are gargantuan. CONSUMER REPORTS tested entrées from major dinner chains last year. We found a chicken-and-noodle meal from Claim Jumper that, with its side dishes, checked out at 3½ pounds and 3,461 calories—more than twice the recommended daily intake for an average-sized, sedentary adult woman.

It's possible, as dieters learn with great effort, to get used to eating a reasonable amount at a restaurant and take the rest home. But our hard-wired instinct, evolved over eons of unreliable food supplies, is to gorge when food is available.

The effect of serving size on modern appetites was ingen-

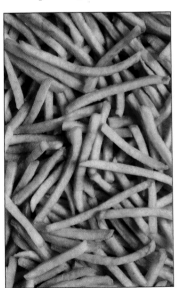

French fries are plentiful and cheap, but sometimes it's better to hold 'em.

iously demonstrated in a study published in the June 2004 *American Journal of Clinical Nutrition* by Tanja Kral, Ph.D., of Penn State, who invited 39 women to eat breakfast, lunch, and dinner in her lab once a week for six weeks. The lunches ranged widely in calorie count and portion size. On the days they drew the higher-calorie, larger-portion lunch, the women ate an average of 56 percent more calories than when they got the lower-calorie, smaller-portion version—even though they reported feeling equally full. And regardless of how many calories they had consumed at lunch, they ate the same amount at dinner.

In another study, published in June 2004 in the *Journal of the American Medical Association*, obese and normal-weight teenagers were taken to a mall fast-food court and allowed to consume as many chicken nuggets, french fries, cookies, and bottles of Coke that they wanted. "Kids consume massive amounts of fast food when provided supersize portions," said one of the researchers, Cara Ebbeling, Ph.D., from Children's Hospital Boston. The normal-weight kids ate an average of 57 percent of their daily caloric requirement at that one sitting; the obese kids ate even more, 67 percent.

POURING ON THE POUNDS

The cheapest calories of all—and the weightiest—may be the ones that come in liquid form. The first year that Americans drank more soda than milk was 1976; they now drink twice as much. Soft drinks displace other, more nutritious beverages. Children ages 6 to 12 who drank 9 ounces or more of soft drinks a day ingested nearly 200 calories per day more than those who didn't, but less milk and fruit juice, according to federal nutrition data analyzed by scientists at the University of Minnesota, reported in an April 1999 issue of the *Journal of the American Medical Association*.

And soft drinks are more available to children and teens than ever before. School systems now have "pouring contracts" with soft-drink companies, which pay fees that can run into millions of dollars for the exclusive right to put vending machines in school buildings and sell their products at school events.

These extra calories are adding up. A two-year study of 548 Massachusetts schoolkids by scientists from Children's Hospital Boston found that for every additional serving of sugar-sweetened drink per day, the risk of obesity rose by 60 percent. The findings were reported in February 2001 in the British medical journal *The Lancet*.

"It may be that the body doesn't compute these calories in the same way; you don't feel full," says Marion Nestle, chair of the nutrition department at New York University.

Researchers at Denmark's Royal Veterinary and Agricultural University demonstrated this phenomenon by giving 21 slightly overweight adults the equivalent of about 40 ounces of sugared drinks a day along with their regular diet; a matched group got the same quantity of artificially sweetened drinks. By the end of the 10-week study, reported in the October 2002 *American Journal of Clinical Nutrition*, the sugar drinkers were consuming nearly 500 calories a day more than they had at the beginning and had gained an average of 3 pounds; the group assigned artificially sweetened drinks was consuming about 100 calories a day less and had lost a bit more than 2 pounds, on average.

The number of recommended calories for most age groups has been cut back because of our increasingly sedentary habits.

SUGAR-COATED ADVICE?

Even as Americans have been consuming ever-larger quantities of sugary, high-fat, and high-calorie drinks and foods, the government's official nutritional advice has steadily

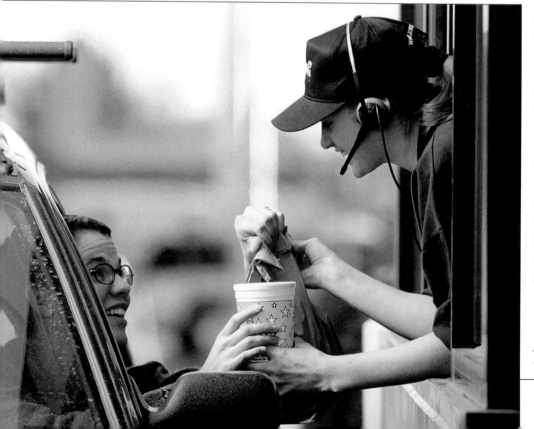

When the convenience of fast food is irresistible, take advantage of the new lower-calorie options.

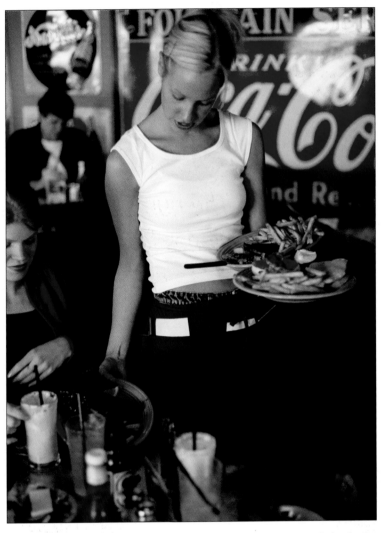

retreated from forthrightly stating that people should consume less of these things.

The 1985 edition of the U.S. Department of Agriculture's *Dietary Guidelines for Americans* advised us to "avoid too much fat, saturated fat, and cholesterol" and to "avoid too much sugar." In the current version, issued in 2000, we aren't told to "avoid" any foods. Instead, the guidelines say, "choose beverages and foods to moderate your intake of sugars" and "choose a diet that is low in saturated fat and cholesterol and moderate in total fat."

Does this seemingly minor change in wording matter? Yes, argues Marion Nestle: "Dietary recommendations can be exploited to sell food products, but they can also turn the public away from entire categories of foods."

The committee of outside nutrition experts assembled to advise the USDA in creating the 2000 dietary recommendations wanted to tell Americans to "go easy on beverages and foods high in added sugars," Nestle reveals in her book, *Food Politics*. But after lobbying by the sugar and grocery industries, the USDA overrode its own appointed experts and came up with the less restrictive wording.

The lobbying continues—openly now. In the spring of 2003, for instance, the sugar industry battled against an upcoming World Health Organization nutrition report that concludes soft drinks are a cause of obesity and recommends that added sugars be restricted to less than 10 percent of caloric intake. Two U.S. senators who co-chair the Senate Sweetener Caucus, Larry E. Craig of Idaho and John Breaux of Louisiana, urged cabinet members to pressure WHO to "cease further promotion" of the report. It came out as scheduled.

The battle over "eat less" advice is likely to continue with the upcoming 2005 revisions of the dietary guidelines as well as the USDA's proposed revision of the familiar Food Guide Pyramid.

The major change from the current edition of the pyramid is a significant cutback in recommended calories for most age groups—a concession to our increasingly sedentary habits. The current guidelines say that "most children" need about 2,200 calories a day; the revised version drops that to 1,200 calories for sedentary girls and 1,400 for sedentary boys under age 9. The current guidelines allow 2,800 calories a day for "very active" women; the revised guidelines peak at 2,400 calories, and then only for women in their 20s who exercise for an hour or more a day.

SUBSIDIZING FATTENING FOODS

Between 1982 and September 2003, the consumer price of fresh fruits and vegetables increased a hefty 127 percent. But the price of fats and oils rose only 57 percent; carbonated soft drinks, 26 percent, and ground beef fattened

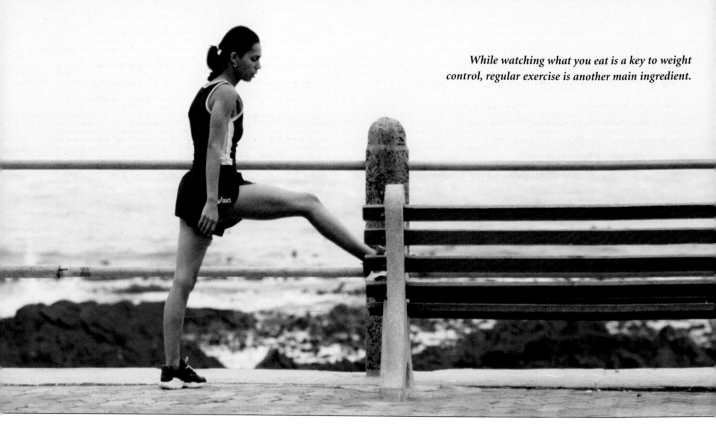

While watching what you eat is a key to weight control, regular exercise is another main ingredient.

on cheap grains, 50 percent. It's no accident that the foods that are making us obese are relatively cheap.

A key reason is that each year about $20 billion of our taxes are spent to subsidize the production of rice, soybeans, sugar, wheat, and—above all—corn. No such subsidy program exists for fruits and vegetables.

The U.S both produces and consumes more corn than any other country. Corn is not only the chief recipient of farm aid, but also the engine behind cheap, high-calorie food in general. It's used directly in tacos and corn chips. It's also the main source of feed for the cattle and chickens whose meat supplies the fast-food industry. It becomes the corn oil that goes into fast-food deep fryers and hydrogenated fats, and it produces the high-fructose corn syrup and other corn sweeteners whose ready availability and startlingly low price have helped fuel the rapid growth in soft-drink consumption.

Soft drinks overwhelmingly use corn syrup, not more expensive cane or beet sugar, as a sweetener. American corn-syrup consumption has multiplied by 40 times in the last 20 years.

Since the New Deal era, farm subsidies were designed to support reasonable prices for farm products by, in effect, paying farmers for not overproducing crops. But starting in 1996, the subsidy system switched over to a simpler plan: For every bushel of subsidized crops they grow, farmers get money from the government. If the market price of the crop drops, not to worry: Subsidy payments increase to make up the difference.

With no check on production and a guaranteed price for their products, farmers naturally produce as much as they can. Oversupply makes the market price go down: Between 1996 and 2000, the price that food manufacturers had to pay for grain fell by nearly half. To compensate, subsidy payments went up to the point where they now constitute, on average, about half of farmers' total income. Since the U.S. dominates world commodity markets, subsidies have also driven down prices in foreign countries and led to repeated clashes over trade policy.

"The money that goes through these programs is captured by cattlemen who get cheap feed, by General Mills who gets cheap grain, and by Monsanto so it can sell more Roundup weed killer," says Harwood Schaffer, a research associate at the Agricultural Policy Analysis Center at the University of Tennessee. "For $2.56, Frito-Lay can buy 56 pounds of corn for making Doritos."

Government food policy is not just an agricultural issue, but also a consumer issue. It's time to think carefully about what can be done to encourage more-healthful eating at both the production and purchasing ends of the food cycle. Some ideas from obesity experts that warrant further investigation include the following:

- Consumers should not be an afterthought in setting agricultural policy. Since our tax dollars pay for both farm subsidies and for obesity in the form of increased public-health expenditures, the government should require health-impact statements from subsidy proposals, much as public-works projects must go through environmental-impact reviews.

- Governments could mandate disclosure of nutritional information on fast-food and chain-restaurant menus.

- More funding could be allocated for marketing the benefits of healthful eating and physical activity. In 2002, the promotional budget for the federal Five A Day program, which encourages consumption of five servings a day of produce, totaled about $12 million, compared to the billions spent promoting snack foods. Some experts propose that a small tax on soft drinks, candy, and other "foods of minimal nutritional value" could be used to fund campaigns to promote better nutrition and more physical activity.

WHAT YOU CAN DO

If you eat reasonable portions of nutritious food at least most of the time, you'll go a long way toward protecting your waistline and your health.

Minimize, don't supersize. At the movies, buy the child-size bag of popcorn—which, despite its name, is probably bigger than the large size of 30 years ago. When the convenience of fast food is irresistible, get a plain burger or grilled chicken sandwich and side salad, if available. Hold the mayo, hold the fries, and go easy on the salad dressing.

Vote with your pocketbook. Patronize restaurants that reveal calorie counts or have healthier choices on the menu. If the portion is oversized, move half of everything to one side of your plate before you begin eating. That's tomorrow's dinner. Or share an entrée, or order only an appetizer and salad.

Fruit juices may be a wiser choice than soft drinks, but they often contain added sugar and lack the nutrients found in whole fruits.

Don't drink sugar. Stay away from sugared sodas or juice drinks with added sugars. Instead, drink water, skim milk, tea, or, when you want a sweet taste, artificially sweetened sodas and juice drinks.

Mind your fruits and veggies. At a restaurant, ask for a double portion of vegetables instead of the starch. Eat a piece of fruit for your afternoon snack instead of visiting the vending machine.

Cook in. The produce industry is offering more vegetables already washed, sliced, and ready to steam, stir-fry, or toss into a salad. It takes just a few minutes to cook a lean chicken breast or piece of fish. If you don't know how, buy a basic cookbook and learn. It isn't difficult.

Keep moving. Regular exercise is vital for maintaining a healthy weight. If you're considering buying exercise equipment, see our buying guides to bicycles (page 70) and treadmills (page 86).

Shop smarter. The label on that 2¾-ounce bag of Ruffles says it's 160 calories. But did you notice that the bag contains "three servings"?

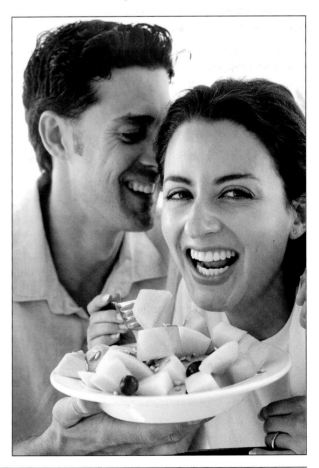

Snacks:
the next generation

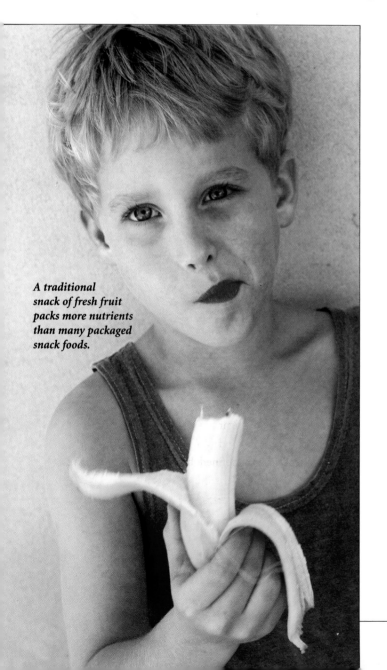

A traditional snack of fresh fruit packs more nutrients than many packaged snack foods.

Honey-wheat Rold Gold pretzels. Natural Ruffles potato chips. Organic…Tostitos? Welcome to the new millennium of snacking, where "natural," "organic," and, most recently, "no trans fat" have succeeded "light" and "fat-free" from the 1990s as the marketing buzzwords for mainstream snack foods.

Salty-snack powerhouse Frito-Lay's Natural line includes seven snacks made either with organic ingredients or without preservatives or artificial colors. The company has also eliminated artery-clogging trans fat from its major brands. Supermarket shelves now burst with those and other earthy-themed snacks, from Good Health Veggie Stix to puffed-rice "Booty" of every flavor from Robert's American Gourmet, an all-natural-snack maker.

Have we entered an era of good-for-you vending-machine goodies? Not exactly. Most "natural" or "organic" snacks, as well as reduced-fat snacks, are still largely bereft of nutrients, and some have even more calories or sodium than the standard versions.

However, many of them do offer modest improvements. Cutting trans fat, found in partially hydrogenated vegetable oil, is a positive step, and organic ingredients generally have fewer pesticides than nonorganic ones. Moreover, foods labeled "natural" may contain fewer or no preservatives or artificial ingredients. And some are at least a bit more nutritious. Consider these examples:

• Robert's American Gourmet Veggie Booty contains less sodium and less fat than most regular crunchy snacks.

• Snyder's of Hanover EatSmart Veggie Crisps supply as much fiber per serving as a slice of whole-wheat bread. However, they contain the same amount of calories as

Old vs. new snacks

Each section of this table lists a traditional version of a snack followed by one or more newer versions.
All serving sizes are 1 ounce; note that single-serving bags from vending machines may exceed those amounts.

Snack	Calories	Total Fat (grams)	Sodium (milligrams)
CHEESE PUFFS			
Cheetos Cheese Flavored Snacks	160	10	350
Cheetos Natural White Cheddar Puffs	170	10	320
CHIPS/CRISPS			
Ruffles Potato Chips	160	10	160
Ruffles Natural Reduced Fat Potato Chips	140	6	210
Glenny's Soy Crisps	110	2	270
Snyder's of Hanover Veggie Crisps	140	7	290
MICROWAVE POPCORN			
Orville Redenbacher's Regular Butter [1]	88	5	137
Orville Redenbacher's Natural Light [1]	50	3	100
PRETZELS			
Snyder's of Hanover Pretzel Sticks	110	1	300
Snyder's of Hanover Organic Oat Bran Pretzel Sticks	120	0	320
TORTILLA CHIPS			
Tostitos 100% White Corn Restaurant Style Tortilla Chips	130	6	80
Tostitos Blue Corn Natural Restaurant Style Tortilla Chips	140	6	110
OTHER			
GeniSoy Soy Nuts Deep Sea Salted	120	4	150
Dry-roasted almonds, salted	166	15	221
Robert's American Gourmet Veggie Booty	140	6	130

[1] Contains trans fat. Note: The FDA's recommended daily maximums for adults, based on a 2,000-calorie diet are total fat, 65 grams, and saturated fat, 20 grams, for sodium, the recommended maximum is 2,400 milligrams, regardless of caloric intake. Chart originally appeared in the March 2004 issue of CONSUMER REPORTS on Health newsletter.

Snyder's regular potato chips, more fat, and about three times the sodium.

• Cheetos Natural White Cheddar Puffs contain slightly less sodium per serving than regular Cheetos—though that's still 13 percent of the recommended daily maximum.

WHAT TO LOOK FOR

If you eat a healthful diet overall, an occasional empty-calorie treat shouldn't do you any harm. But follow these tips:

• **Know your fats.** Look for products that don't contain trans fat or, if that's not labeled, no partially hydrogenated oil.

• **Consider baked or reduced-fat snacks.** The baked versions are almost always lower in fat, and the reduced-fat or light ones have at least 25 percent less fat than the originals. However, those "lighter" options may be only mar-ginally lower in calories. And some have more sodium.

• **Check sodium and sugar.** In general, chips have the least salt; pretzels have the most. Flavored varieties of any snack tend to have significantly more sodium than regular versions. Low-fat or otherwise "improved" products often add extra salt or sugar.

• **Be careful with "natural."** Unlike "organic," the claim "natural" is not defined by the Food and Drug Administration, so check the ingredients list.

• **Find value-added options.** Snacks that include fiber, protein, or both are likely to keep you fuller longer than mere carbohydrates, and they offer some nutritional benefit. Nuts or soy snacks pack plenty of protein and fiber; treats that list a whole grain (such as whole wheat) or bran as the first ingredient should provide at least 2 grams of fiber per serving.

Index

Index

Photo Credits

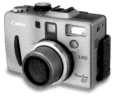
Digital Cameras

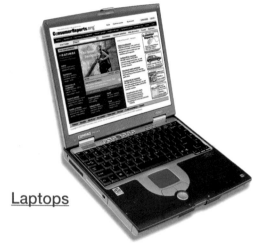
Laptops

KIRKWOOD

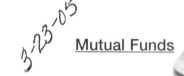
Vacuum Cleaners

TRY OUR SITE FREE FOR 30 DAYS!

3-23-05

Mutual Funds

Cars

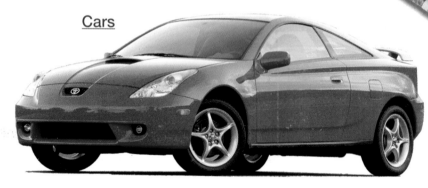

ConsumerReports.org

Get even more of what you want from CONSUMER REPORTS:

Quick access to the latest Ratings, interactive tools to help you find the right products, side-by-side comparisons, e-Ratings, PDA downloads and more!

Go to <u>ConsumerReports.org/cr/free30</u> for your free trial!

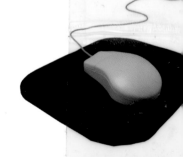